The elenpilates™
Stockpile Textbook

The elenpilates™ Stockpile Textbook

Connecting Joe Pilates' exercises between technique and practice

Elaine Mary Dutton

iUniverse, Inc.
New York Lincoln Shanghai

The elenpilates™ Stockpile Textbook
Connecting Joe Pilates' exercises between technique and practice

iUniverse, Inc.

For information address:
iUniverse, Inc.
2021 Pine Lake Road, Suite 100
Lincoln, NE 68512
www.iuniverse.com

ISBN: 0-595-31925-4

Printed in the United States of America

ACKNOWLEDGMENTS

The task in compiling the Elenpilates™ Stockpiles Textbook required the motivation that I acquired from the talented, patient, understanding, and concerning distinguished health and fitness individuals that I still have the privilege and honor to work with.

- I am deeply grateful and very proud of my fitness clients, the posing models for the exercises contained within. They are not health instructors nor trained athletes, but dedicated ladies with only a three-month training session they acquired with me within the Pilates technique. I hope their dedication shown in the photographs encourages you as they encouraged me to continue:

Privé Fitness Club (Piraeus)
Katerina Patiniotou, Eleni Velmahou, Maria Dritsa

Sprinter's Fitness Club (Peristeri)
Angelica Labrou, Olga Kotroni, Ourania Harakopoulou

Sprinter's Fitness Club (Ano Patissia)
Labrini Psihogiou, Aphrodite Andriolatou, Irene Skorda, Rallou Liberi, Lilian Christouli, Jenny Georgana

Some names may not have been added due to publication deadlines

- Within the field of Health & Fitness in Greece, I owe my prime establishment to a distinguished educationalist and mentor, Prof. Panagiotis Sidiropoulos, from Dynamiki Zoi S.A.—Universal Studios. My eternal gratitude to this gentleman.
- My appreciative position to the production team at iUniverse Publishers in giving me the opportunity and in undertaking this project.
- My admiration goes to John Spencer Ellis, MBA, Ed.D, and President of the National Endurance & Sports Training Association (NESTA) for his unbelievable confidence in me over the years.
- I express my thanks to the professional team of Class 2001, 2002 and 2003 at the Graduate Aerobic & Fitness School (GR.A.F.T.S.) for their organization and contribution to the world of fitness that sparkled upon me.
- My recognition goes to the photographer, Mr. Panos Panagiotides, who had the kindness to authorize, for this project, the submission of my portrait photograph on the back cover.

- And finally, I would like to thank the persons whom hold this textbook in their hands; you are my most important critic and value your opinion. I welcome your comments. You may email me at: info@elenpilates.com or visit my website at www.elenpilates.com.

Thank you all!

Elaine Mary Dutton (2004)

CONTENTS

A Brief History of Joe Pilates

Joseph Hubertus Pilates was born near Düsseldorf (Germany) and though as a child he grew up suffering from rickets, asthma and rheumatic fever, he managed at his young age to overcome his health problems and began to study anatomy, Eastern and Western bodyworks that included yoga, Zen, and ancient Greek and Roman regimens.

At the age of fourteen he became a successful boxer, gymnast, skier and diver. He was even asked to model for anatomy charts then set out for England during World War I but was captivated in a camp for enemy aliens. During his time in camp, he put to use his knowledge to help rehabilitate bedridden patients, using bedsprings as equipment. Today, such equipment is largely seen embedded into fitness clubs, health studios, dancing schools, and clinics.

In 1925, after the war, he returned to Germany and was offered to train the New German Army, but decided to head for America instead. It was on this journey that he met his future wife, Clara. They both opened a gym in New York City close to a number of ballet and dance schools that captivated the dancing legions such as Martha Graham, Jerome Robbins and George Balanchine who all incorporated the Pilates principles into their lessons.

Pilates died in a fire outbreak in 1967, at the age of eighty-seven. His wife Clara continued to teach and run the studio until her death 10 years later.

HOW TO USE THIS TEXTBOOK

Each stockpile is presented with detailed instructions on the exercises within the stockpiles. Where there is a photograph showing the exercise, it is marked with (Fig) and its sequential number within the exercise.

There are Pilates baby stockpiles and also Athletic Tai-Chi stockpiles that can be chosen in case you do not have too much time and need a swift workout. You can also add any of the standing series exercises to your stockpile workouts that you will find at the end of the textbook.

It is essential that all stockpiles be preceded with Stockpile Workout 1, which is the initial warm-up stockpile in order to initiate blood circulation. You can also end your workouts with Stockpile Workout 12, which is the cool-down or utilize it when you are feeling any tension during a hard day and just want to relax.

Each stockpile targets specific areas of the body. You may choose any stockpile to workout on, depending on your time frame and in the comfort of your home. No equipment is necessary, except for a mat or a blanket to protect the spine whilst doing these exercises. You may also need to use a soft pillow, especially if you are a beginner, to protect the neck flexors from straining whilst in the C-shape spine position (*See 'The Hundred' exercise Fig.1*).

After some time these neck flexors will get stronger and you will no longer need the pillow to assist you. Wherever a pillow is necessary, it has been indicated in the exercise accordingly.

Each exercise contains a section on the benefits and what to look out for. Should you have any doubts whatsoever if the exercise is suitable for you, please consult your physician or physical therapy practitioner before undertaking the exercise.

I must stress that taking these exercises one step at a time will be well worth your moment in time. Always begin with the basic levels, wherever appropriately stated in the exercise, before you venture to higher levels. It will make you too uncomfortable to try higher levels before you have given your body a chance to strengthen. (*See Labrini struggling for levels beyond comfort in stockpile workout 4, The Leg Pull Front Fig.1.*)

The following technique postures are used extensively throughout the exercises. Refer back to these pages for reference whenever doubtful.

The Pilates Stance (Fig.1)

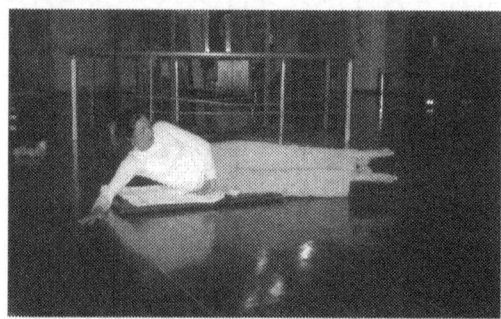

This is the first position in ballet: Bring the heels together and turn your thighs out then point the toes (plantar flexion). Imagine a zip in the inner thighs from your heels up to the top of the leg that needs to be zipped up to eliminate any light passing through the legs. This leg posture aims to target the inner thighs.

The C-Shape spine (Fig.2)

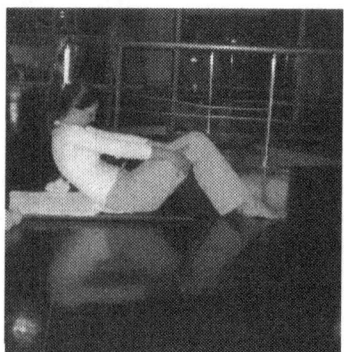

This is the "scoop" the navel to spine technique: Your spine curls back into the letter C of the English alphabet. Imagine holding a small tennis ball between the chin and the sternum (chest). This arrangement initiates the powerhouse, the five lumbar and the five sacrum vertebrae, to protect your lower back.

The Charlie Chaplin Stance (Fig.3)

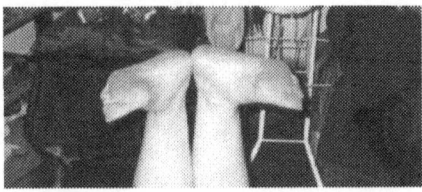

Remember how Charlie Chaplin used to place his feet when standing? Well, this is it. It requires the same leg technique as the Pilates Stance (Fig.1) first position in ballet, but the only difference is that the toes are not pointed but flexed (dorsi flexion).

For a satisfied flexed position throughout the exercises, press through the heels as though they are guiding the movements with toes facing towards the knees, and you will feel the entire leg-work, especially the front thighs (quadriceps) and an amazing stretch on the back of the thighs (hamstrings).

Shoulders

Always try to eliminate the shrugging of the shoulders in the exercises to release tension in the neck. Tension is caused from the Trapezius muscle, a large diamond-shaped muscle where the upper fibers tend to over-work.

NOTES

Child Pose

After each stockpile or in between exercises, you need to give your spine a rest and relax in the Child Pose position. Whenever you feel a need to relax do this relaxing pose:

1. From a table top position sit the hips back onto your heels
   Important Note:
   Should you have delicate knees just add a soft pillow between the knee joints as you sit on the heels to eliminate any additional tension
2. Let the chest sink down towards the floor
3. Stretch the arms forward with hands on the floor and lower the forehead to the mat

Yoga Mudra

The yoga Mudra helps relieve headaches, migraines, opens the heart center (4th chakra), kindles the crown chakra and stretches the back and arms. It is worth a try at the end of your stockpile workout if you feel comfortable with this asana. Should you feel any dizziness during the pose leave it out of your workout:

1. From a table top position bend the elbows so your torso lowers to the floor
2. Rest the crown of your head on the mat
   Important Note:
   Should you feel dizzy at this point just rest back onto your heels and slowly build that spine vertebrae by vertebrae against an imaginary wall. Remain in this position (Japanese style) till you feel the dizziness has gone and do not continue with the yoga Mudra
3. Try to keep the crown of the head on the mat and not the forehead or the hairline
4. If you feel comfortable enough, interlace your fingers behind you and stretch the arms to the ceiling
5. Breath and hold for 2-6 breaths
6. Release the arms then lower your hips to the heels into child pose

The Butterfly

During some exercises you may feel that your back needs some relaxation. You can do The Butterfly pose to relax the whole back and relieve those Trigger points* by stretching the Trapezius muscles:

1. Sit on the floor and bring your legs towards you to connect the inner sole together with knees looking to the sides
2. Grasp gently around the ankles then curl the upper body forward allowing the head to fall forward over your bent legs
3. Release the shoulders towards the floor and remain here for 12 seconds

*Trigger Points are those confined small areas in muscles that are tangible knots or lumps.

NOTES

GLOSSARY

Technique

Articulating the spine: Imagine peeling the spine off the mat vertebrae by vertebrae to initiate flexibility throughout length

Stockpile: A chain of Pilates mat work exercises in a block

Scoop the belly: Your spine curls back into the letter C of the English alphabet. Imagine holding a small tennis ball between the chin and the sternum (chest). This arrangement initiates the powerhouse, the 5 lumbar and the 5 sacrum vertebrae, to protect your lower back

Long neck: When the head is tucked in and chin holding the imaginary tennis ball, the neck lengthens with the crown looking towards the ceiling

Crown: Top of the head that looks at the ceiling when in a standing position

Pilates Stance: When the feet are with pointed toes in first position ballet

Charlie Chaplin Stance: When the feet are flexed in first position ballet

Zip up inner thighs: Imagine a zip between your legs from the ankles up to the highest part of your inner thighs. Zip up to eliminate any light passing between the legs

NOTES

Anatomical Terms

Medial: Towards the mainline of the body

Lateral: Away from the mainline of the body

Anterior: Front of the body

Posterior: Back of the body

Inferior: Away from the head

Plantar flexion: Pointed toes

Dorsi flexion: Toes brought upwards

Uniarticulate: Muscle crossing one joint

Biarticulate: Muscle crossing two joints

Extension: Increasing the joint

Hyperextension: Increasing the joint beyond normal

Flexion: Decreasing the joint

Rotation: A turn around the long axis

Circumduction: A 360° rotation

Proximal attachment: Origin of the muscle

Distal attachment: Insertion of the muscle

Supination: Palm faced upwards

Pronation: Palm faced downwards

Prone Position: Lying on your stomach

Supine Position: Lying on your back

90-degree angle: (a) When lying on the floor with knees bent (b) when the legs are stretched towards the ceiling (c) when the elbows are bent and in line with the ribs without touching the mat

45-degree angle: When lying on the floor and the legs are in a diagonal line from the body

35-degree angle: When lying on your back with head tucked in and the shoulders are at a 35-degree angle from the mat (C-shape spine)

NOTES

Muscles

Hamstrings: Back side of the thigh

Quadriceps: Front side of the thigh

Abdominal area: Stomach muscles

Abduction: Away from the body

Adduction: Towards the body

Buttocks: The gluteus muscles

Eccentric phase: Shortening of the muscle

Concentric phase: Lengthening of the muscle

Isotonic contraction: This is when a muscle shortens in length and the origin of the muscle comes closer to the insertion of the muscle. Imagine this contraction when you do the curl up in a supine position (lying on your back). The Rectus Abdominis flexes the trunk as it curls up and is in conflict from the weight of the body due to gravity. Now imagine this contraction when you do the dive forward from a standing position. The Rectus Abdominis flexes the trunk (that is what it does) in the dive however it is not conflicting from the weight of the body as gravity is causing the trunk to fall forward

Isometric contraction: This is when the muscle length stays the same but the force changes. Imagine this contraction when in The Isometric exercise as you are holding your body up without movement and there is no muscle contraction; the length stays the same however the muscles are working against gravity.

Types of stretches:

Static—recommended without risk of injury. This is a stretch that is held to the point of comfort for approximately 10-30 seconds

Ballistic—not recommended due to increase of possible injury and soreness to the muscle fiber. This bouncing stretch should be eliminated from your Pilates workout

PNF (Propioceptive Neuromuscular Facilitation—used in physical therapy where a stretch is used immediately after a muscle contraction. It is used in The Mermaid exercise

Dynamic—a controlled stretch that has movement but without the bouncing effect. It is used in the Spine Twists

Spinal deformity: Spinal deformity means abnormality in the curves of the spine taking us to the most frequently seen in adolescence: Scoliosis. It is a lateral of sideways curvature of the spine that turns on its axis like a corkscrew. The cause of idiopathic scoliosis, a common form, is unknown causing shoulder, trunk and waistline asymmetry.

The Spine: The human spine consists of 33 vertebrae and is examined from top to bottom
- 7 cervical vertebrae (neck region) that connects the head to the thorax
- 12 thoracic vertebrae (chest region) that is circular when an abnormal curve is seen and is termed as Kyphosis, which means "humpback". These curves produce the normal rounding of the shoulder that we all have to some degree, and curves of 20 to 40 degrees are considered normal. For curves over 40 degrees, an exercise program is requested. Surgery is not performed to correct Kyphosis unless the curve goes beyond 75 degrees
- 5 lumbar vertebrae (back & lower back region) that articulates with the sacrum. If there is an exaggeration of this curve it is termed Lordosis
- 5 sacrum vertebrae (lower back region) located between the two Ilia
- 4 coccyx vertebrae (tail bone region)

NOTES

NOTES

WORKOUT STOCKPILES

WARM-UP
Stockpile Workout 1
- The Hundred
- Windmill Arms
- Role Up/Down
- Tilt Back Torso

ABDOMINALS
Stockpile Workout 2
- Single Leg Stretch
- Crisscross
- Straight Leg Open/Close
- Double Straight Leg Stretch
- Double Leg Stretch
- Beach Ball
- Walking Roof

SPINE/ABDOMINALS
Stockpile Workout 3
- Pelvic Shoulder Bridge
- Roll Over
- Corkscrew
- Scissors

ABDOMINALS
Stockpile Workout 4
- The Ball
- The Teasers
- The Teaser & Circle
- Leg Pull Front
- Oblique Tilt Back

BODY WORKOUT
Stockpile Workout 5
- The Crab
- The Boomerang
- Rocking Chair
- The Can-Can
- The Mermaids
- Side Isometrics

LEGS/HIPS/BUTTOCKS
Stockpile Workout 6
- Side Lifts
- All Side Leg Lifts (5)
- Inner Thigh Lifts
- Inside Leg Circle
- Archer's Legs

BACK (KYPHOSIS/LORDOSIS)
Stockpile Workout 7
- The Ballerinas

BUTTOCKS/LEGS
Stockpile Workout 8
- Butt Chopper
- The Pigeon (Yoga Asana)

ARMS/SCOLIOSIS/ABDOMINALS
Stockpile Workout 9
- The Seal
- Rowing
- Spine Twists (Scoliosis)
- The Saw (Scoliosis)
- Russian Curl
- Spine Stretch Forward

BODY WORKOUTS/NECK
Stockpile Workout 10
- The Arrow
- The Diamond
- Neck Roll
- Planks
- Leg Pull Back
- The Swan Dive

BODY WORKOUTS/LEGS
Stockpile Workout 11
    Push-Up
    Cat Legs
    The Bear (Yoga Asana)
    Swimming
    Breast Stroke

COOL-DOWN
Stockpile Workout 12
    Upside Down Table
    Shoulder Lifts
    Dead Zone

PILATES BABY STOCKPILES

Baby Stockpile 1
Neck Roll
Swan Dive

Baby Stockpile 2
    Hip Circles
    Can-Can

Baby Stockpile 3
Side Isometric Level 1
Chest Expansion

Baby Stockpile 4
    Chest Expansion
    The Mermaid

Baby Stockpile 5
Pilates Lunges
Curtsey Lunges

Baby Stockpile 6
    Scissors I, II

Baby Stockpile 7
Ballerina One
The Ball

STANDING SERIES

Biceps I, II
The Bug
The Boxer
Shaving the Head

Triceps
Chest Expansion
The Zipper
Arm Circles

Standing Wall Peeling the Spine
Standing Cool Down

Standing Chair

ATHLETIC TAI-CHI STOCKPILES

Abduction
Repulse the Monkey

Parting Horse's Rein
Horse Stance

STOCKPILE WORKOUTS

**Important Note: All Stockpiles should begin with Stockpile Workout 1

<u>Stockpile Workout 1</u>

The Hundred

The Windmill Arms

Role Up/Down

Tilt Back Torso

The Hundred

<u>Technique (Fig.1)</u>

1.   Lie in a supine position (on your back) with legs bent at a 90-degree angle so your soles are in contact with the floor

2.   Bring your arms by your side lengthening the fingers and slightly bend at the elbows with palms facing the floor. This will protect the shoulder in its socket

3.   Begin by raising the head off the mat and imagine you are holding a small tennis ball between your chin and sternum (chest). This will allow for a long neck. The shoulders are now in a 35-degree angle off the mat

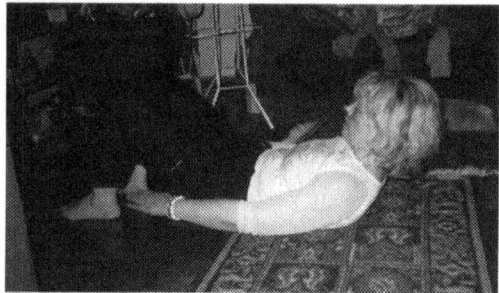

Fig. 1

<u>Workout</u>

4.   Begin pumping your arms close to the floor with a small range of motion

5.   Inhale for 5 counts, exhale for 5 counts, inhale for 5 counts, exhale for 5 counts

6.   Raise your legs towards your chest and continue to keep them bent (Fig.2)

7.   Inhale for 5 counts, exhale for 5 counts

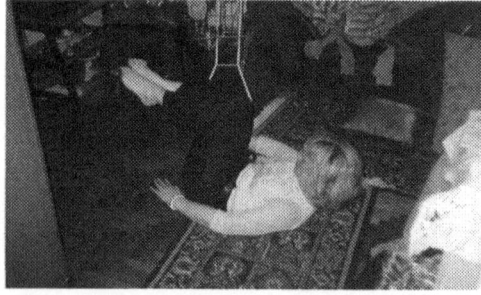

Fig. 2

8.   Stretch your legs towards the ceiling in a Pilates Stance. This will have the legs in a 90-degree angle (Fig. 3)

9.   Inhale for 5 counts, exhale for 5 counts

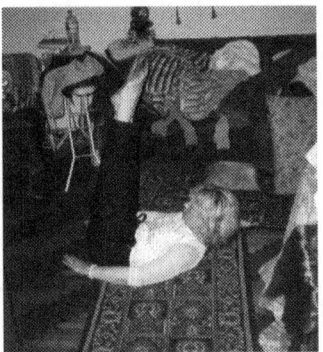

Fig. 3

10. Slightly lower your stretched out legs diagonally in front of you
11. This will now have the legs in a 45-degree angle with toes in line with the forehead
12. Inhale for 5 counts, exhale for 5 counts, inhale for 5 counts, exhale for 5 counts
     <u>Important note:</u>
     If you feel tension in your neck, use a soft pillow to rest your head on. Should you feel that your lower back is lifting from the floor then re position those straight legs to stretch once again towards the ceiling and continue
13. Stretch your legs again towards the ceiling (90-degree angle)
14. Inhale for 5 counts, exhale for 5 counts; bend your legs again towards the chest
15. Inhale for 5 counts exhale for 5 counts. Bring your legs once again to the mat so your soles are positioned on the floor. Inhale for 5 counts, exhale for 5 counts
16. Rest your head and shoulders to the mat

<u>Benefits</u>
The Hundred allows for a complete body warm-up and initiates blood circulation. It is a classical Pilates exercise that can be done in sections according to comfort as shown in the photographs.

<u>Watchfulness</u>
Keep in mind that you always need to scoop the belly in towards the spine. Do not hold your breath; a continuous inhale of 5 counts and exhale of 5 counts should be maintained throughout the exercise to complete one hundred breaths, hence the name of the exercise.

Try to keep your shoulders pressed away from your ears in order to eliminate the shrugging of shoulders and to provide for a long neck. If your neck feels uncomfortable, you can always use a pillow to rest your head throughout the exercise until your deep neck flexors become accustomed to the motion and begin to strengthen with time.

You have just completed The Hundred exercise. Good work! Continue with The Windmill Arms when you feel comfortable to continue.

**Important Note: All Stockpiles should begin with Stockpile Workout 1

<u>Stockpile Workout 1</u>

The Hundred

The Windmill Arms

Role Up/Down

Tilt Back Torso

The Windmill Arms

<u>Technique</u>

1. Lie in a supine position (on your back) with legs bent and soles on the floor
2. This will allow for the legs to be in a 90-degree angle
3. Stretch one arm next to your ear whilst the other arm stretches by your thigh. Palms are faced inwards with long fingers
4. Begin by raising the head off the mat and imagine you are holding a small tennis ball between your chin and sternum (chest). This will allow for a long neck. The shoulders are now in a 35-degree angle off the mat

    <u>Important note:</u>

    If you feel tension in your neck use a soft pillow to rest your head on

    <u>Workout</u>

5. Switch the arms like a windmill through the air
6. Imagine scissoring and cutting through the air always having the switch come back to arm position with one arm next to the ear and the other by your side
7. Switch 2 times (right, left), bring both arms by your side and try to raise the torso higher just an inch
8. Hold this position then slowly lower the upper body and arms to rest on the mat
9. Repeat the entire sequence 3 times

Benefits
The windmill arms allows for a complete body warm-up, improves co-ordination, stabilizes the shoulder blades, and initiates the abdominal area.

The abdominals (abdomen) are four abdominal muscles in partitions:
1. The Transverse Abdominal muscles are the deepest of the four that force the air from the lungs, hence the exhale acquired whilst lifting is initiated in abdominal exercises
2. The Rectus Abdominal muscle functions to flex the trunk. We can see this movement done when the body is in the C-shape spine position on the mat
3. Internal and External Obliques work to rotate the trunk

Watchfulness
Keep in mind that you always need to scoop the belly in towards the spine. Do not hold your breath; a continuous inhale of 5 counts and exhale of 5 counts should be maintained throughout the exercise.

Try to keep your shoulders pressed away from your ears in order to eliminate shrugging and produce a long neck. Keep those arms long as they scissor through the air. If your neck feels uncomfortable, you can always use a pillow to rest your head throughout the exercise until your neck flexors become accustomed to the motion and begin to strengthen with time.

You have just completed The Windmill Arms exercise. Good work! Continue with Role Up/Down when you feel comfortable to continue.

**Important Note: All Stockpiles should begin with Stockpile Workout 1
<u>Stockpile Workout 1</u>
The Hundred
The Windmill Arms
Role Up/Down
Tilt Back Torso

Role Up/Down

<u>Technique—Level 1</u>

1. Lie in a supine position (on your back) with legs stretched out in a Pilates Stance. Point the toes
2. Take your arms and stretch them over your head to rest on the floor
3. Squeeze the buttocks to help you when you begin to curl up
    <u>Workout—Level 1</u>
4. Begin to peel the spine off the mat vertebrae by vertebrae (Fig. 1) starting with the hands, head, shoulders, upper back and when you have finally peeled the spine off the mat take the torso into a forward Pilates bend (Fig. 2)

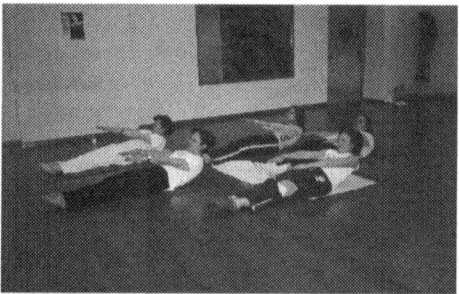

Fig. 1

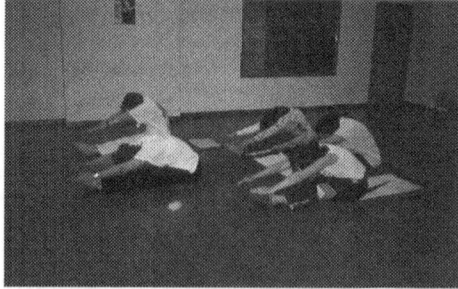

Fig. 2

5. This is a position where your torso is stretched forward over your legs and arms stretched next to the ears
    <u>Important note:</u>
    If your lower back feels uncomfortable in the Pilates bend, just bend the knees to alleviate any additional tension
6. Begin to slowly uncurl and back down towards the mat
7. Repeat this sequence 3-5 times

Technique—Level 2

8.   Lie in a supine position (on your back) with legs stretched out to hip distance. Flex the feet and bring your hands behind your head and interlace your fingers. Keep the elbows out and looking to the sides

9.   Squeeze the buttocks that will help you curl your spine up from the mat

Workout—Level 2

10. Begin to peel the spine off the mat vertebrae by vertebrae starting with the head, shoulders, upper back and when you have finally peeled the spine off the mat take the torso into a forward Pilates bend

11. This is a position where your torso is stretched forward over your legs and arms behind your head with interlaced fingers. Keep the elbows out and looking to the sides (this placement reduces Scoliosis)

Important note:

If your lower back feels uncomfortable in the Pilates bend, just bend the knees to alleviate any additional tension

12. When you finally peel up into a forward Pilates bend, slowly build that spine to a sitting position and imagine your spine is resting against a wall

13. Begin to slowly uncurl and back down towards the mat. Repeat 3-5 times

Benefits

The Role Up/Down articulates the spine and also initiates the abdominal area.

The abdominals (abdomen) are four abdominal muscles in partitions:

1.   The Transverse Abdominal muscles are the deepest of the four that force the air from the lungs, hence the exhale acquired whilst lifting is initiated in abdominal exercises

2.   The Rectus Abdominal muscle functions to flex the trunk. We can see this movement done when the body is in the C-shape spine position on the mat

3.   Internal and External Obliques work to rotate the trunk

Watchfulness

Keep in mind that you always need to scoop the belly in towards the spine as you peel the spine off the floor. Do not hold your breath; a continuous inhale of 5 counts and exhale of 5 counts should be maintained throughout the exercise.

If you feel uncomfortable, you can always release those arms and grasp the sides of your legs to help you peel off the floor until your abdominal muscles become accustomed to the motion and begin to strengthen.

You have just completed the Role Up/Down exercise. Good work! Continue with Tilt Back Torso when you feel comfortable to continue.

**Important Note: All Stockpiles should begin with Stockpile Workout 1

Stockpile Workout 1

The Hundred

The Windmill Arms

Role Up/Down

Tilt Back Torso

Tilt Back Torso

Technique

1. Lie in a supine position (on your back) with legs stretched out to hip distance. Flex the feet
2. Bring your hands behind your head and interlace your fingers. Keep the elbows out and looking to the sides
3. Squeeze the buttocks that will help you curl your spine up from the mat

Workout

4. Begin to peel the spine off the mat vertebrae by vertebrae starting with the head, shoulders, upper back and when you have finally peeled the spine off the mat take the torso into a forward Pilates bend
5. This is a position where your torso is stretched forward over your legs and arms behind your head with interlaced fingers. Keep the elbows out and looking to the sides (this placement reduces Scoliosis)

Important note:

If your lower back feels uncomfortable in the Pilates bend, just bend the knees to alleviate any additional tension
6. When you finally peel up into a forward Pilates bend, slowly build that spine to a sitting position and imagine your spine is resting against a wall
7. Slightly tilt the torso back (keeping that straight spine) to where you feel comfortable
8. Scoop into the C-shape spine bringing those elbows in
9. Slowly roll that spine back towards the mat vertebrae by vertebrae
10. Repeat the sequence 3-5 times

Benefits
The Tilt Back Torso articulates and helps to elongate the spine with initiating the abdominal area.

The abdominals (abdomen) are four abdominal muscles in partitions:
1. The Transverse Abdominal muscles are the deepest of the four that force the air from the lungs, hence the exhale acquired whilst lifting is initiated in abdominal exercises
2. The Rectus Abdominal muscle functions to flex the trunk. We can see this movement done when the body is in the C-shape spine position on the mat
3. Internal and External Obliques work to rotate the trunk

Watchfulness
Keep in mind that you always need to scoop the belly in towards the spine as you peel the spine off the floor. Do not hold your breath; a continuous inhale of 5 counts and exhale of 5 counts should be maintained throughout the exercise.

Try to keep your elbows back looking to the sides without pulling on your head to initiate the peel off. If you feel uncomfortable, you can always release those arms and grasp the sides of your legs to help you peel off the floor until your abdominal muscles become accustomed to the motion and begin to strengthen.

You have just completed the Tilt Torso Back exercise and Stockpile 1. Good work!

All of the following Stockpiles can be done in independent order. Choose the one that most suits you and remember, always begin your workouts with Stockpile 1. Enjoy!

IMPROVEMENT RECORD STOCKPILE WORKOUT 1

The Hundred

The Windmill Arms

IMPROVEMENT RECORD STOCKPILE WORKOUT 1

Role Up/Down

Tilt Back Torso

**Important Note: All Stockpiles should begin with Stockpile Workout 1
Stockpile Workout 2
Single Leg Stretch
Crisscross
Straight Leg Open/Close
Double Straight Leg Stretch
Double Leg Stretch
Beach Ball
Walking Roof

Single Leg Stretch

Technique

1. Lie in a supine position (on your back) with legs bent at a 90-degree angle so your soles are in contact with the floor
2. Raise the legs towards your chest and keep them bent
3. Bring the arms to hug the right leg just below the knee and stretch the left leg in front of you. This will bring the straight leg to a 45-degree diagonal angle
4. Begin by raising the head off the mat and imagine you are holding a small tennis ball between your chin and sternum (chest). This will allow for a long neck. The shoulders are now in a 35-degree angle off the mat (Fig.1)

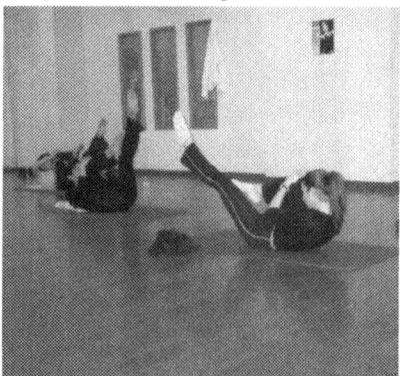

Fig. 1

Important note:

If you feel uncomfortable or feel that your lower back is lifting from the floor then re position that stretched out leg to the ceiling. This will bring the leg to a 90-degree angle straight up. You may also need to use a soft pillow, especially if you are a beginner, to protect the neck flexors from straining whilst in this position. After some time these neck flexors will get stronger and you will no longer need the pillow to assist you.

Workout

5. Pulse the right leg towards you for 2 small pulses
6. Switch legs: Bring the arms to hug the left leg just below the knee and stretch the right leg in front of you. This will bring the straight leg to a 45-degree diagonal angle

7. Continue to switch legs till you do a repetition of 10 switches
8. Remember to exhale with each leg switch

Benefits
The Single Leg Stretch initiates the abdominal area.

The abdominals (abdomen) are four abdominal muscles in partitions:
1. The Transverse Abdominal muscles are the deepest of the four that force the air from the lungs, hence the exhale acquired whilst lifting is initiated in abdominal exercises
2. The Rectus Abdominal muscle functions to flex the trunk. We can see this movement done when the body is in the C-shape spine position on the mat
3. Internal and External Obliques work to rotate the trunk

Watchfulness
Keep in mind that you always need to scoop the belly in towards the spine. Do not hold your breath; a continuous exhale to each leg switch should be maintained throughout the exercise.

Try to keep your elbows open looking to the sides without pulling on your bent leg to keep you up. If you feel uncomfortable, you can always rest your head on pillow or do the exercise with legs in a 90-degree angle towards the ceiling until your abdominal muscles and neck flexors become accustomed to the motion and begin to strengthen.

You have just completed the Single Leg Stretch exercise. Good work! Continue with the Crisscross when you feel comfortable to continue.

**Important Note: All Stockpiles should begin with Stockpile Workout 1

<u>Stockpile Workout 2</u>

Single Leg Stretch

Crisscross

Straight Leg Open/Close

Double Straight Leg Stretch

Double Leg Stretch

Beach Ball

Walking Roof

Crisscross

<u>Technique</u>

1. Lie in a supine position (on your back) with legs bent at a 90-degree angle so your soles are in contact with the floor
2. Raise the legs towards your chest and keep the right leg bent as you stretch the left leg in front of you. This will bring the straight leg to a 45-degree diagonal angle
3. Bring your hands behind your head and interlace the fingers. Keep the elbows back looking to the sides
4. Begin by raising the head off the mat and imagine you are holding a small tennis ball between your chin and sternum (chest). This will allow for a long neck. The shoulders are now in a 35-degree angle off the mat

<u>Important note:</u>

If you feel uncomfortable or feel that your lower back is lifting from the floor then re position that stretched out leg to the ceiling. This will bring the leg to a 90-degree angle straight up. If you feel that you are pulling on your head to keep you up you may also need to use a soft pillow, especially if you are a beginner, to protect the neck flexors from straining whilst in this position. After some time these neck flexors will get stronger and you will no longer need the pillow to assist you

<u>Workout</u>

5. Twist the torso to the right. Try to see if you can touch the right knee with the left elbow (Fig. 1). Look behind at the right elbow without allowing it to touch the floor

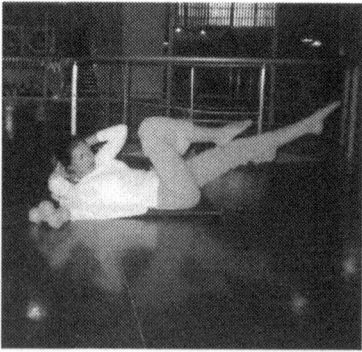

Fig. 1

6.   Twist to the other side: Try to see if you can touch the left knee with the right elbow Look behind at the left elbow without allowing it to touch the floor
7.   Keep switching sides till you do a repetition of 5 switches
8.   When you have accomplished this slow twist, try to see if you can speed up the exercise without losing the technique for another 5 twists each side
9.   If you feel that the technique is lost abandon the faster twists till your body gets stronger and more familiar with the exercise. Do not allow the hips to lift from the mat; stabilize them avoiding the rocking motion
10. Exhale with each switch

Benefits
The Crisscross initiates the abdominal area, especially the Obliques.

The abdominals (abdomen) are four abdominal muscles in partitions:
1.   The Transverse Abdominal muscles are the deepest of the four that force the air from the lungs, hence the exhale acquired whilst lifting is initiated in abdominal exercises
2.   The Rectus Abdominal muscle functions to flex the trunk. We can see this movement done when the body is in the C-shape spine position on the mat
3.   Internal and External Obliques work to rotate the trunk

When the trunk rotates, united with flexion as in the Crisscross, there is a simultaneous effect of the internal oblique of one side and the external oblique of the other side.

Watchfulness
Keep in mind that you always need to scoop the belly in towards the spine. Do not hold your breath; a continuous exhale to each switch should be maintained throughout the exercise.

Try to keep your elbows open looking to the sides without pulling on your head to keep you up. If you feel uncomfortable, you can always rest your head on pillow or do the exercise with legs in a 90-degree angle towards the ceiling until your abdominal muscles and neck flexors become accustomed to the motion and begin to strengthen.

You have just completed the Crisscross exercise. Good work! Continue with the Straight Leg Open/Close when you feel comfortable to continue.

**Important Note: All Stockpiles should begin with Stockpile Workout 1
<u>Stockpile Workout 2</u>
Single Leg Stretch
Crisscross
Straight Leg Open/Close
Double Straight Leg Stretch
Double Leg Stretch
Beach Ball
Walking Roof

Straight Leg Open/Close
<u>Technique</u>
1. Lie in a supine position (on your back) with legs bent at a 90-degree angle so your soles are in contact with the floor
2. Raise those legs towards your chest then stretch them towards the ceiling in a Pilates Stance. This will have the legs in a 90-degree angle
3. Begin by raising the head off the mat and imagine you are holding a small tennis ball between your chin and sternum (chest). This will allow for a long neck. The shoulders are now in a 35-degree angle off the mat
4. Bring your hands behind your head and interlace the fingers. Keep the elbows back looking to the sides
   <u>Workout</u>
5. Lower those stretched legs in front of you. This will bring the legs to a 45-degree diagonal angle
   <u>Important note:</u>
   If you feel uncomfortable or feel that your lower back is lifting from the floor then re position those stretched out legs to the ceiling. This will bring the leg to a 90-degree angle straight up. If you feel that you are pulling on your head to keep you up you may also need to use a soft pillow, especially if you are a beginner, to protect the neck flexors from straining whilst in this position. After some time these neck flexors will get stronger and you will no longer need the pillow to assist you
6. Begin to open and close the legs for 5 counts. Keep the opening to shoulder width
7. When done, take the legs back towards the ceiling, bend the legs towards the chest and end with legs bent and feet in contact with the floor
8. Rest the shoulders and head on the mat

Benefits

The Straight Leg Open/Close initiates the abdominal area.

The abdominals (abdomen) are four abdominal muscles in partitions:

1. The Transverse Abdominal muscles are the deepest of the four that force the air from the lungs, hence the exhale acquired whilst lifting is initiated in abdominal exercises

2. The Rectus Abdominal muscle functions to flex the trunk. We can see this movement done when the body is in the C-shape spine position on the mat

3. Internal and External Obliques work to rotate the trunk

Watchfulness

Keep in mind that you always need to scoop the belly in towards the spine. Do not hold your breath; a continuous inhale on the open movement and exhale on the closing movement should be maintained throughout the exercise.

Try to keep your elbows open looking to the sides without pulling on your head to keep you up. If you feel uncomfortable, you can always rest your head on a pillow or do the exercise with legs in a 90-degree angle towards the ceiling until your abdominal muscles and neck flexors become accustomed to the motion and begin to strengthen.

You have just completed the Straight Leg Open/Close exercise. Good work! Continue with the Double Straight Leg Stretch when you feel comfortable to continue.

**Important Note: All Stockpiles should begin with Stockpile Workout 1
<u>Stockpile Workout 2</u>
Single Leg Stretch
Crisscross
Straight Leg Open/Close
Double Straight Leg Stretch
Double Leg Stretch
Beach Ball
Walking Roof

Double Straight Leg Stretch

<u>Technique</u>

1. Lie in a supine position (on your back) with legs bent at a 90-degree angle so your soles are in contact with the floor
2. Raise those legs towards your chest then stretch them towards the ceiling in a Pilates Stance. This will have the legs in a 90-degree angle
3. Begin by raising the head off the mat and imagine you are holding a small tennis ball between your chin and sternum (chest). This will allow for a long neck. The shoulders are now in a 35-degree angle off the mat
4. Bring your hands behind your head and interlace the fingers. Keep the elbows back looking to the sides

<u>Workout</u>

5. Lower those stretched legs in front of you. This will bring the legs to a 45-degree diagonal angle. Inhale
6. Raise the legs once again towards the ceiling. Exhale

<u>Important note:</u>

If you feel uncomfortable or feel that your lower back is lifting from the floor then re position those stretched out legs to the ceiling and continue doing a smaller range of motion instead. If you feel that you are pulling on your head to keep you up you may also need to use a soft pillow, especially if you are a beginner, to protect the neck flexors from straining whilst in this position. After some time these neck flexors will get stronger and you will no longer need the pillow to assist you

7. Repeat the sequence 4 more times
8. Bend the legs towards the chest and end with legs bent and feet in contact with the floor
9. Rest the shoulders and head on the mat

Benefits

The Double Straight Leg Stretch initiates the abdominal area.

The abdominals (abdomen) are four abdominal muscles in partitions:

1.   The Transverse Abdominal muscles are the deepest of the four that force the air from the lungs, hence the exhale acquired whilst lifting is initiated in abdominal exercises

2.   The Rectus Abdominal muscle functions to flex the trunk. We can see this movement done when the body is in the C-shape spine position on the mat

3.   Internal and External Obliques work to rotate the trunk

Watchfulness

Keep in mind that you always need to scoop the belly in towards the spine. Do not hold your breath; a continuous inhale on the down movement and exhale on the up movement should be maintained throughout the exercise.

Try to keep your elbows open looking to the sides without pulling on your head to keep you up. If you feel uncomfortable, you can always rest your head on a pillow until your neck flexors become accustomed to the motion and begin to strengthen.

You have just completed the Double Straight Leg Stretch exercise. Good work! Continue with the Double Leg Stretch when you feel comfortable to continue.

**Important Note: All Stockpiles should begin with Stockpile Workout 1

<u>Stockpile Workout 2</u>

Single Leg Stretch

Crisscross

Straight Leg Open/Close

Double Straight Leg Stretch

Double Leg Stretch

Beach Ball

Walking Roof

Double Leg Stretch

<u>Technique</u>

1. Lie in a supine position (on your back) with legs bent at a 90-degree angle so your soles are in contact with the floor
2. Raise those legs towards your chest
3. Begin by raising the head off the mat and imagine you are holding a small tennis ball between your chin and sternum (chest). This will allow for a long neck. The shoulders are now in a 35-degree angle off the mat
4. Bring your hands to clasp over the shins; keep the elbows out looking to the sides
   <u>Workout</u>
5. Take those arms, stretch them overhead keeping them near your ears. Circle the arms around you and bring them to lightly clasp over the shins again. Try not to let the circle movement disrupt your technique; keep the shoulders 35-degrees off the mat. Repeat this sequence 3 times
   <u>Important note:</u>
   If you feel uncomfortable or feel that your lower back is lifting from the floor then re position those stretched out legs to the ceiling and continue. If you feel that your neck is straining you may also need to use a soft pillow, especially if you are a beginner, to protect the neck flexors from straining whilst in this position. After some time these neck flexors will get stronger and you will no longer need the pillow to assist you
6. Now lets add the legs. As you stretch the arms out bringing them next to the ears (Fig. 1) stretch the legs simultaneously in front of you to a 45-degree diagonal angle
7. Circle the arms around you and bring them back to lightly clasp over the shins as you bring back the legs to their original position
8. Repeat this sequence 3 times then rest the shoulders, head and legs onto the mat

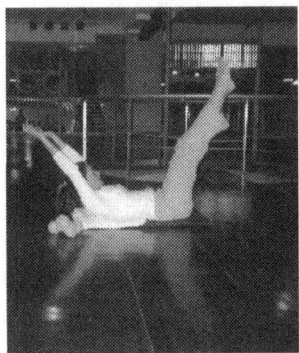

Fig. 1

<u>Benefits</u>
The Double Leg Stretch initiates the abdominal area.

The abdominals (abdomen) are four abdominal muscles in partitions:
1. The Transverse Abdominal muscles are the deepest of the four that force the air from the lungs, hence the exhale acquired whilst lifting is initiated in abdominal exercises
2. The Rectus Abdominal muscle functions to flex the trunk. We can see this movement done when the body is in the C-shape spine position on the mat
3. Internal and External Obliques work to rotate the trunk

<u>Watchfulness</u>
Keep in mind that you always need to scoop the belly in towards the spine. Do not hold your breath; a continuous inhale on the stretch out movement and exhale on the in movement should be maintained throughout the exercise.

If you feel uncomfortable, you can always rest your head on a pillow until your neck flexors become accustomed to the motion and begin to strengthen.

You have just completed the Double Leg Stretch exercise. Good work! Continue with the Beach Ball when you feel comfortable to continue.

**Important Note: All Stockpiles should begin with Stockpile Workout 1

<u>Stockpile Workout 2</u>

Single Leg Stretch

Crisscross

Straight Leg Open/Close

Double Straight Leg Stretch

Double Leg Stretch

Beach Ball

Walking Roof

Beach Ball

<u>Technique</u>

1. Lie in a supine position (on your back) with legs bent at a 90-degree angle so your soles are in contact with the floor
2. Raise those legs towards your chest then stretch them towards the ceiling in a Pilates Stance. This will have the legs in a 90-degree angle
3. Begin by raising the head off the mat and imagine you are holding a small tennis ball between your chin and sternum (chest). This will allow for a long neck. The shoulders are now in a 35-degree angle off the mat
4. Bring your hands behind your head and interlace the fingers. Keep the elbows back looking to the sides

   <u>Workout</u>
5. Bring the legs to hip width and imagine you are holding between your feet (between the inside of the calves) a beach ball
6. Twist that imaginary beach ball you have between your legs to the left then to the right

   <u>Important note:</u>

   Should you feel uncomfortable with straight legs, keep them slightly bent until the hamstrings get more stronger. You may also need to use a soft pillow, especially if you are a beginner, to protect the neck flexors from straining whilst in this position. After some time these neck flexors will get stronger and you will no longer need the pillow to assist you
7. Close the legs, bend them towards your chest, and take the legs to the floor again and rest the shoulders and head onto the mat
8. Repeat the sequence 5 times

Benefits
The Beach Ball initiates the abdominal area.

The abdominals (abdomen) are four abdominal muscles in partitions:

1. The Transverse Abdominal muscles are the deepest of the four that force the air from the lungs, hence the exhale acquired whilst lifting is initiated in abdominal exercises
2. The Rectus Abdominal muscle functions to flex the trunk. We can see this movement done when the body is in the C-shape spine position on the mat
3. Internal and External Obliques work to rotate the trunk

Watchfulness
Do not hold your breath; a continuous inhale on the turning of the ball to the right and exhale on the turning of the ball to the left movement should be maintained throughout the exercise. If you feel uncomfortable, you can always rest your head on a pillow until your neck flexors become accustomed to the motion and begin to strengthen.

You have just completed the Beach Ball exercise. Good work! Continue with the Walking Roof when you feel comfortable to continue.

**Important Note: All Stockpiles should begin with Stockpile Workout 1

<u>Stockpile Workout 2</u>

Single Leg Stretch

Crisscross

Straight Leg Open/Close

Double Straight Leg Stretch

Double Leg Stretch

Beach Ball

Walking Roof

Walking Roof

<u>Technique</u>

1. Lie in a supine position (on your back) with legs bent at a 90-degree angle so your soles are in contact with the floor
2. Raise those legs towards your chest then stretch them towards the ceiling in a Pilates Stance. This will have the legs in a 90-degree angle
3. Keep the upper body resting on the mat and palms facing down on the floor

    <u>Workout</u>
4. Flex those feet and begin to do small walking paces as if you were walking on the roof

    <u>Important note:</u>

    Should you feel uncomfortable with straight legs, keep them slightly bent until the hamstrings get more stronger
5. Do about 10 paces before you bend the legs into your chest again and to the floor

Benefits
The Walking Roof initiates the abdominal area especially the lower section and strengthens the hips.

The abdominals (abdomen) are four abdominal muscles in partitions:
1. The Transverse Abdominal muscles are the deepest of the four that force the air from the lungs, hence the exhale acquired whilst lifting is initiated in abdominal exercises
2. The Rectus Abdominal muscle functions to flex the trunk. We can see this movement done when the body is in the C-shape spine position on the mat
3. Internal and External Obliques work to rotate the trunk

Watchfulness
Do not hold your breath; a continuous inhale on one pace and exhale on the other pace should be maintained throughout the exercise.

You have just completed the Walking Roof exercise and Stockpile 2. Good work!

IMPROVEMENT RECORD STOCKPILE WORKOUT 2

Single Leg Stretch

Crisscross

Straight Leg Open/Close

Double Straight Leg Stretch

IMPROVEMENT RECORD STOCKPILE WORKOUT 2

Double Leg Stretch

Beach Ball

Walking Roof

**Important Note: All Stockpiles should begin with Stockpile Workout 1

<u>Stockpile Workout 3</u>

Pelvic Shoulder Bridge

Roll Over

Corkscrew

Scissors

Pelvic Shoulder Bridge

<u>Technique</u>

1. Lie in a supine position (on your back) with legs bent at a 90-degree angle so your soles are in contact with the floor

2. Keep the torso on the mat with hands by your sides and palms facing down

    <u>Workout</u>

3. Begin to slowly peel the spine off the mat beginning with the pelvis area

4. Peel the coccyx (tail bone), sacrum (lower back) off the mat vertebrae by vertebrae and have your bent legs and buttocks support your weight

5. Hold the body up with the spine in one straight line. Try not to add too much weight on those shoulders

6. Slowly begin to peel the spine back to the mat vertebrae by vertebrae until your tail bone and pelvis are once again resting against the mat

7. Repeat this sequence 3 times

Benefits

The Pelvic Shoulder Bridge articulates the spine, initiates the gluteus muscles, thighs and neck.

Watchfulness

Do not hold your breath; a continuous inhale on the peeling off the spine from the mat and exhale on the return of the spine towards the mat should be maintained throughout the exercise.

Keep most of the weight relaxed on the shoulders as you squeeze the buttocks to hold you up and keep the spine in one straight line against gravity.

You have just completed the Pelvic Shoulder Bridge exercise. Good work! Continue with the Roll Over when you feel comfortable to continue.

**Important Note: All Stockpiles should begin with Stockpile Workout 1
<u>Stockpile Workout 3</u>
Pelvic Shoulder Bridge
Roll Over
Corkscrew
Scissors

Roll Over

Eliminate this exercise if you have any spinal problems such as a slipped disk

<u>Technique</u>
1.   Lie in a supine position (on your back) with legs in a Pilates Stance stretched out in contact with the floor
2.   Keep the hands by your sides with palms facing the floor
<u>Workout</u>
3.   Begin to raise the legs and peel the spine off the mat vertebrae by vertebrae till those legs come over your head (Fig. 1)
4.   Open the legs to hip distance and flex the feet
5.   Now slowly roll back down onto the mat vertebrae by vertebrae
<u>Important note:</u>
Eliminate the above exercise if you have any spinal problems such as a slipped disk and do this version: If you feel too uncomfortable with the legs stretched, try keeping them bent and only raise the pelvis off the floor a few inches to initiate the abdominal area
6.   Repeat this sequence 3 times and then do it again but reversing the action of the feet
7.   Lie in a supine position (on your back) with legs at hip distance and feet flexed
8.   Begin to raise the legs and peel the spine off the mat vertebrae by vertebrae till those legs are over your head
9.   Close the legs in a Pilates Stance and slowly roll back down onto the mat vertebrae by vertebrae
10.   Repeat this sequence 3 times

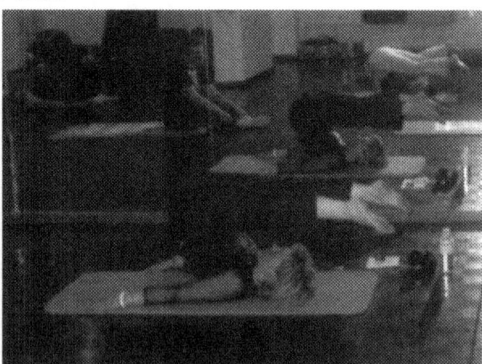

Fig. 1

<u>Benefits</u>
The Roll Over articulates the spine and initiates the abdominal area.

The abdominals (abdomen) are four abdominal muscles in partitions:
1.   The Transverse Abdominal muscles are the deepest of the four that force the air from the lungs, hence the exhale acquired whilst lifting is initiated in abdominal exercises
2.   The Rectus Abdominal muscle functions to flex the trunk. We can see this movement done when the body is in the C-shape spine position on the mat
3.   Internal and External Obliques work to rotate the trunk

<u>Watchfulness</u>
Do not hold your breath; a continuous inhale on peeling off the mat and exhale on the return of the spine towards the mat should be maintained throughout the exercise.

Press the palms onto the floor when peeling the spine off the mat to help. Eliminate this exercise with straight legs if you have any spinal problems such as a slipped disk and do it with the legs bent and raising only the pelvis from the mat.

You have just completed the Roll Over exercise. Good work! Continue with the Corkscrew when you feel comfortable to continue.

**Important Note: All Stockpiles should begin with Stockpile Workout 1
<u>Stockpile Workout 3</u>
Pelvic Shoulder Bridge
Roll Over
Corkscrew
Scissors

Corkscrew

Eliminate Level 2 of this exercise if you have any spinal problems such as a slipped disk and do Level 1 version.

<u>Technique—Level 1</u>
1. Lie in a supine position (on your back) and bend those legs into your chest to a 90-degree angle
2. Keep the torso on the mat with hands by your sides and palms looking down
<u>Workout—Level 1</u>
3. Take the hips towards the right and peel the right side of the spine off the mat vertebrae by vertebrae till the pelvis raises
4. Slowly roll the pelvis back down to the mat
5. Take the hips towards the left and peel the left side of the spine off the mat vertebrae by vertebrae till the pelvis raises
6. Slowly roll the pelvis back down to the mat
7. Repeat the sequence 3 times to each side of the spine
<u>Technique—Level 2</u>
8. Lie in a supine position (on your back) and legs in a Pilates Stance stretched out in front of you.
9. Keep the torso on the mat with hands by your sides and palms looking down
<u>Workout—Level 2</u>
10. Take the hips towards the right and peel the right side of the spine off the mat vertebrae by vertebrae till those legs are over your head
11. Slowly roll back down on the right side of the spine onto the mat vertebrae by vertebrae
12. Take the hips towards the left and peel the left side of the spine off the mat vertebrae by vertebrae till those legs are over your head
13. Slowly roll back down on the left side of the spine onto the mat vertebrae by vertebrae
14. Repeat the sequence on each side of the spine 3 times
<u>Important note:</u>
Eliminate Level 2 of this exercise if you have any spinal problems such as a slipped disk and do Level 1 version.

Benefits

The Corkscrew articulates the left and right side of the spine (Sacrospinalis). If there is a weakness on one side, it usually causes a sideway bend. Should both sides be weak, it results in the slouching posture.

Watchfulness

Do not hold your breath; a continuous inhale on the peeling off the mat and exhale on the return of the spine towards the mat should be maintained throughout the exercise. Press the palms onto the floor when peeling the spine off the mat to help.

Eliminate this exercise with straight legs (Level 2) if you have any spinal problems such as a slipped disk and do it with the legs bent (Level 1) and raising only the pelvis from the mat

You have just completed the Corkscrew exercise. Good work! Continue with the Scissors when you feel comfortable to continue.

**Important Note: All Stockpiles should begin with Stockpile Workout 1
<u>Stockpile Workout 3</u>
Pelvic Shoulder Bridge
Roll Over
Corkscrew
Scissors

Scissors

<u>Technique</u>

1. Lie in a supine position (on your back) and stretch your legs towards the ceiling in a Pilates Stance. This will have the legs in a 90-degree angle
2. Begin by raising the head off the mat and imagine you are holding a small tennis ball between your chin and sternum (chest). This will allow for a long neck. The shoulders are now in a 35-degree angle off the mat
3. Hold above the knee or around the calf and take one leg towards your face and the other leg towards the floor without letting the leg touch the mat
   <u>Workout</u>
4. Pulse for 2 counts the leg towards your face and the other leg simultaneously pulses for 2 counts towards the floor. (Fig. 1)
5. Switch legs. Inhale on one switch and exhale on the other switch
6. Repeat the sequence and alternate for 10 switches with each leg
   <u>Important note:</u>
   Try to keep your shoulders pressed away from your ears in order to eliminate the shrugging of shoulders and to provide for a long neck. If your neck feels uncomfortable, you can always use a pillow to rest your head throughout the exercise until your neck flexors become accustomed to the motion and begin to strengthen with time. Do not worry if you feel uncomfortable in stretching those legs. Keep them slightly bent and grasp behind the leg above the knee for the exercise, till your hamstrings become stronger

<u>Benefits</u>
The Scissors initiates the abdominal area and stretches the hamstrings.

The abdominals (abdomen) are four abdominal muscles in partitions:
1.   The Transverse Abdominal muscles are the deepest of the four that force the air from the lungs, hence the exhale acquired whilst lifting is initiated in abdominal exercises
2.   The Rectus Abdominal muscle functions to flex the trunk. We can see this movement done when the body is in the C-shape spine position on the mat
3.   Internal and External Obliques work to rotate the trunk

The hamstrings flex the knee and extend the thigh. The Scissors exercise stretches the hamstrings, as too tight hamstrings can lead to spine problems. This can be noticed when one sits on the floor with legs stretched out in front.

Difficulty arises to sit on the Ischial Tuberosities (sitting bones) and Lordosis (inward curve of the lower back) begins to initiate. It is advisable to eliminate any additional tension by sitting on a pillow to bring the pelvis higher than the legs.

<u>Watchfulness</u>
Keep in mind that you always need to scoop the belly in towards the spine. Do not hold your breath; a continuous inhale on one leg switch and exhale on the other leg switch should be maintained throughout the exercise.

You have just completed the Scissors exercise and Stockpile 3. Good work!

Fig. 1

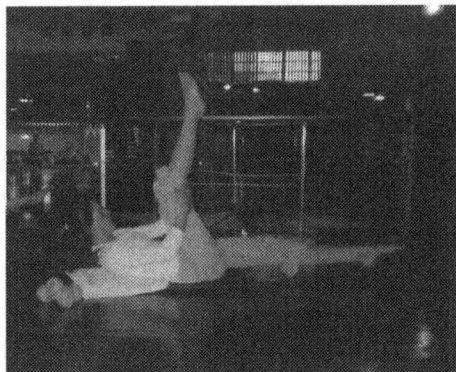

IMPROVEMENT RECORD STOCKPILE WORKOUT 3

Pelvic Shoulder Bridge

Roll Over

IMPROVEMENT RECORD STOCKPILE WORKOUT 3

Corkscrew

Scissors

**Important Note: All Stockpiles should begin with Stockpile Workout 1

<u>Stockpile Workout 4</u>

The Ball

The Teaser

The Teaser & Circle

Leg Pull Front

Oblique Tilt Back

The Ball

<u>Technique</u>

1. Sit on the edge of your mat with your legs bent to the chest and gently grasp your shins
2. Tilt back slightly to balance on your sit bones

<u>Workout</u>

3. Keep your head in and elbows out looking to the sides whilst you begin to roll onto the spine vertebrae by vertebrae then roll back up like a ball
4. Repeat the ball exercise for 5 rolls

<u>Important note:</u>

Stop the roll of the spine at the shoulder blades and never onto the neck area

Benefits
The Ball allows for a complete massage to the spine.

Watchfulness
Keep in mind that you always need to scoop the belly in towards the spine. Do not hold your breath; a continuous inhale of rolling down and exhale of rolling up should be maintained throughout the exercise.

Try to keep your shoulders pressed away from your ears in order to eliminate the shrugging of shoulders. Keep those elbows looking to the sides. Stop the roll of the spine at the shoulder blades and never onto the neck area.

You have just completed The Ball exercise. Good work! Continue with The Teaser when you feel comfortable to continue.

**Important Note: All Stockpiles should begin with Stockpile Workout 1

Stockpile Workout 4

The Ball

The Teaser

The Teaser & Circle

Leg Pull Front

Oblique Tilt Back

The Teaser

Level 1

1. Lie in a supine position (on your back) with legs bent at a 90-degree angle so your soles are in contact with the floor
2. Stretch the arms overhead
3. Bring the arms forward and begin to peel the spine off the mat vertebrae by vertebrae till you feel your abdominal area engage
4. Slowly roll back down to the mat vertebrae by vertebrae
Repeat this 3 times

Level 2

5. Lie in a supine position (on your back) with legs bent at a 90-degree angle so your soles are in contact with the floor
6. Stretch the arms overhead
7. Keep the right leg bent with the sole flat on the floor and stretch the left leg forward to the height of the bent leg
8. Begin to bring the arms forward and peel the spine off the mat vertebrae by vertebrae till you feel your abdominal area engage
9. Slowly roll back to the mat vertebrae by vertebrae.
10. Repeat this 3 times with each leg

Level 3

11. Bend both legs into your chest and grasp behind the thighs to roll up into a sitting position
12. Slightly tilt back to sit on your sitting bones with legs bent. This will give the legs a 90-degree angle
13. Grasp under the thighs above the knees
14. Raise the legs so that the toes are slightly higher than knee height
15. Keep the elbows open looking to the sides; connect the shoulder blades and slide them down your spine. Remain in Level 3 for 3 counts then go to level 4

Level 4

16. Release the legs and stretch the arms to your side. (Fig. 1) Remain in Level 4 for 3 counts then go to level 5

Level 5

17. Stretch the legs forward in a Pilates Stance with the arms stretched up beside your ears. Remain in Level 5 for 3 counts—imagine forming a perfect V

<u>Benefits</u>
The Teaser allows for a complete initiation of the abdominal area and body workout.

The abdominals (abdomen) are four abdominal muscles in partitions:
1.   The Transverse Abdominal muscles are the deepest of the four that force the air from the lungs, hence the exhale acquired whilst lifting is initiated in abdominal exercises
2.   Rectus Abdominal muscle functions to flex the trunk. We can see this movement done when the body is in the C-shape spine position on the mat
3.   Internal and External Obliques work to rotate the trunk

<u>Watchfulness</u>
Keep in mind that you always need to scoop the belly in towards the spine. Do not hold your breath.

Try to keep your shoulders pressed away from your ears in order to eliminate the shrugging of shoulders. Keep those elbows looking to the sides when the hands are grasping under the thighs above the knees.

Do not attempt levels 2, 3, 4, and 5 till your body is familiar with level 1.

You have just completed The Teaser exercise. Good work! Continue with The Teaser & Circle when you feel comfortable to continue.

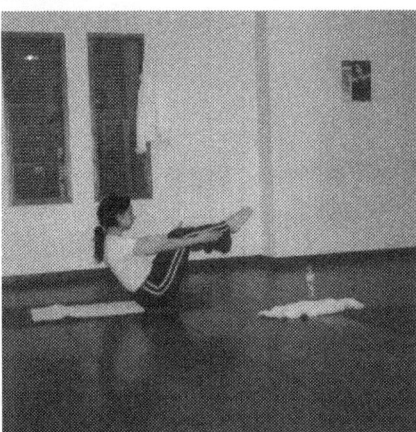

Fig. 1

**Important Note: All Stockpiles should begin with Stockpile Workout 1

<u>Stockpile Workout 4</u>

The Ball

The Teasers

The Teaser & Circle

Leg Pull Front

Oblique Tilt Back

The Teaser & Circle

<u>Technique</u>

1. Sit on your sitting bones and bend your knees grasping under the thighs above the knee joint. This will bring the legs in a 90-degree angle

2. Slightly tilt back to obtain balance and raise the legs so that the toes are slightly higher than knee height

3. Keep the elbows open looking to the sides; connect the shoulder blades and slide them down your spine

<u>Workout</u>

4. Now stretch the arms in front of you and circle them to the right whilst you circle the bent legs to the left. Keep the range of motion small

5. Repeat this sequence 3 times

6. Now circle the arms to the left whilst you circle the legs to the right. Keep the range of motion small

7. Repeat this sequence 3 times

Benefits
The Teaser & Circle allows for a complete initiation of the abdominal area and body workout.

The abdominals (abdomen) are four abdominal muscles in partitions:
1. The Transverse Abdominal muscles are the deepest of the four that force the air from the lungs, hence the exhale acquired whilst lifting is initiated in abdominal exercises
2. The Rectus Abdominal muscle functions to flex the trunk. We can see this movement done when the body is in the C-shape spine position on the mat
3. Internal and External Obliques work to rotate the trunk

Watchfulness
Keep in mind that you always need to scoop the belly in towards the spine. Do not hold your breath; a continuous inhale of one circle and exhale of an opposite circle should be maintained throughout the exercise.

Try to keep your shoulders pressed away from your ears in order to eliminate the shrugging of shoulders. Keep those elbows looking to the sides when the hands are grasping under the thighs above the knees.

You have just completed The Teaser & Circle exercise. Good work! Continue with The Leg Pull Front when you feel comfortable to continue.

**Important Note: All Stockpiles should begin with Stockpile Workout 1

<u>Stockpile Workout 4</u>

The Ball

The Teasers

The Teaser & Circle

Leg Pull Front

Oblique Tilt Back

Leg Pull Front

<u>Technique</u>

1. Sit up and imagine your spine is against an imaginary wall. Take your hands behind you to support your upper body
2. Bend your knees at a 90-degree angle so your soles are in contact with the floor
   <u>Workout—Level 1</u>
3. Begin to raise the pelvis to bring the front body in one straight line with the knees. This is a table top position
4. Raise the right leg with pointed toes to the height of your bent leg, flex the foot and return the leg to the mat
5. Repeat the leg raise with alternating foot from flex to pointed toes 3 times before changing to the other leg. If you want to challenge your body do level 2
   <u>Important note:</u>
   Do not push your progress. Do level 2 only when you have exercised level 1 for some duration
   <u>Technique—Level 2</u>
6. Sit up and imagine your spine is against an imaginary wall. Take your hands behind you to support your upper body. Stretch your legs in front of you in a Pilates Stance
   <u>Workout—Level 2</u>
7. Begin to raise the pelvis to bring the front of the body in a diagonal line with the feet
8. Raise the right leg with pointed toes to the height it is most comfortable, flex the foot and return the leg to the mat (Fig. 1)

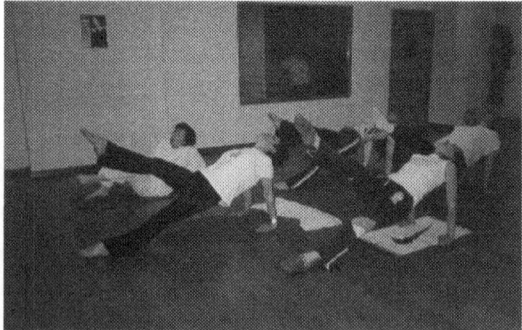

Fig. 1

9. Repeat the leg raise with alternating foot from flex to pointed toes 3 times before changing to the other leg

Benefits
The Leg Pull Front allows for a complete body workout.

Watchfulness
Do not hold your breath; a continuous inhale of leg lift and exhale of one leg lowering should be maintained throughout the exercise. Try to keep your weight from drooping down into the shoulders.

You have just completed The Leg Pull Front exercise. Good work! Continue with The Oblique Tilt Back when you feel comfortable to continue.

**Important Note: All Stockpiles should begin with Stockpile Workout 1

<u>Stockpile Workout 4</u>

The Ball

The Teaser

The Teaser & Circle

Leg Pull Front

Oblique Tilt Back

Oblique Tilt Back

<u>Technique</u>

1.   Lie in a supine position (on your back) with legs stretched out before you in a Pilates Stance
2.   Bring your hands behind your head and interlace your fingers
3.   Keep the elbows back looking to the sides; squeeze the buttocks to help you curl up

<u>Workout</u>

4.   Begin to peel the spine off the mat vertebrae by vertebrae

<u>Important note:</u>

If you feel too uncomfortable, slightly bend the knees or bring the elbows in to help you peel the spine off the mat without pulling on your head to help you up

5.   When you finally peel up into a forward Pilates bend, slowly re build that spine to a sitting position and imagine your spine is straight up against an imaginary wall

<u>Important note:</u>

If you peeled up with elbows in, once you get into the forward Pilates bend take those elbows back again looking to the sides

6.   Bring the arms to fold in front of your chest
7.   Slightly tilt the torso back to where you feel comfortable. Squeezing your buttocks will help you lower further (Fig. 1)

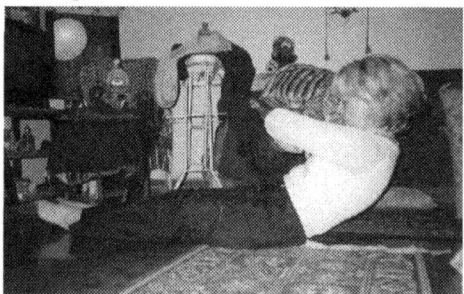

Fig. 1

8.   Twist the torso to the left, swing the left arm to look back with the twist (Fig. 2)

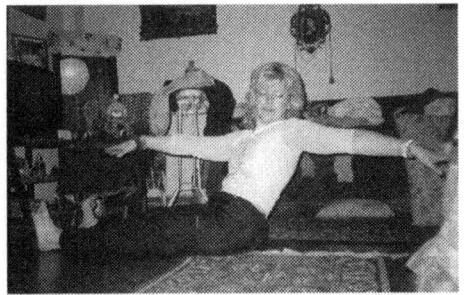

Fig. 2

9. Twist the torso forward again folding the arms in front of your chest. Change sides
10. Twist the torso to the right, swing the right arm to look back with the twist
11. Twist the torso forward again folding the arms in front of your chest
12. Re build that spine to a sitting position and imagine your spine is straight up against an imaginary wall
13. Scoop into a C-shape spine and re peel that spine back towards the mat vertebrae by vertebrae keeping the arms folded in front of the chest
14. Repeat the sequence 3-5 times

<u>Benefits</u>
The Oblique Tilt Back articulates and helps to elongate the spine and also initiates the oblique area.

The abdominals (abdomen) are four abdominal muscles in partitions:
1. The Transverse Abdominal muscles are the deepest of the four that force the air from the lungs, hence the exhale acquired whilst lifting is initiated in abdominal exercises
2. The Rectus Abdominal muscle functions to flex the trunk. We can see this movement done when the body is in the C-shape spine position on the mat
3. Internal and External Obliques work to rotate the trunk

<u>Watchfulness</u>
Keep in mind that you always need to scoop the belly in towards the spine as you peel the spine off the floor. Do not hold your breath; a continuous inhale of one twist and exhale of the opposite twist should be maintained throughout the exercise.

If you feel uncomfortable, you can always release those arms and grasp the sides of your legs to help you peel off the floor until your abdominal muscles become accustomed to the motion and begin to strengthen.

You have just completed the Oblique Tilt Torso exercise and Stockpile 4. Good work!

IMPROVEMENT RECORD STOCKPILE WORKOUT 4

The Ball

The Teaser

The Teaser & Circle

IMPROVEMENT RECORD STOCKPILE WORKOUT 4

Leg Pull Front

Oblique Tilt Back

**Important Note: All Stockpiles should begin with Stockpile Workout 1

<u>Stockpile Workout 5</u>

The Crab

The Boomerang

Rocking Chair

The Can-Can

The Mermaids

Side Isometrics

The Crab

<u>Technique</u>

1. Sit on the edge of your mat with your legs bent to the chest
2. Pass the arms through the inside of the legs so that the palms rest on the outside of the ankles
3. Tilt back slightly to balance on your sit bones (Fig. 1)

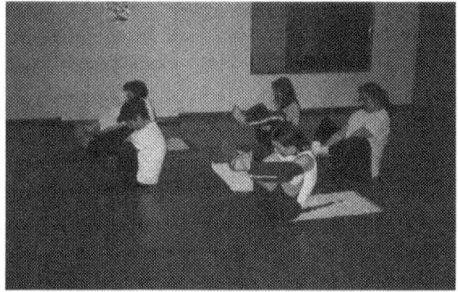

Fig. 1

<u>Workout</u>

4. Roll onto the spine vertebrae by vertebrae then roll back up like a ball (Fig. 2)

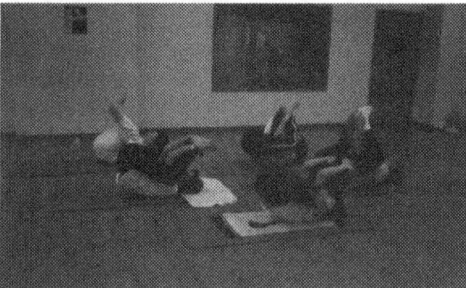

Fig. 2

5. Repeat the sequence for 5 rolls

<u>Important note:</u>

Keep your head gently tucked in and heels close to the buttocks. Imagine forming the shape of a ball. Stop the roll of the spine at the shoulder blades and never onto the neck area

<u>Benefits</u>
The Crab allows for a complete massage to the spinal column. It is a variation of The Ball.

<u>Watchfulness</u>
Keep in mind that you always need to scoop the belly in towards the spine. Do not hold your breath; a continuous inhale of rolling down and exhale of rolling up should be maintained throughout the exercise.

Try to keep your shoulders pressed away from your ears in order to eliminate the shrugging of shoulders. Stop the roll of the spine at the shoulder blades and never onto the neck area.

You have just completed The Crab exercise. Good work! Continue with The Boomerang when you feel comfortable to continue.

**Important Note: All Stockpiles should begin with Stockpile Workout 1
<u>Stockpile Workout 5</u>
The Crab
The Boomerang
Rocking Chair
The Can-Can
The Mermaids
Side Isometrics

The Boomerang

Eliminate this exercise entirely if you have any spinal problems such as a slipped disk

The Boomerang is a Stockpile of the Teaser and the Roll Over

<u>Technique</u>
1. Sit tall and imagine your spine is resting against an imaginary wall
2. Straighten the legs on the floor in front of you then cross the right ankle over the left
    <u>Workout</u>
3. Begin to roll back bringing the legs overhead just as in the Roll Over exercise
4. Open and close the legs re crossing. This time your left ankle crosses over the right
5. Roll back up into a V shape sitting position with legs stretched out in front of you at a 45-degree angle and arms stretched up by your ears
6. Lean forward till your legs touch the floor; take the arms in a circle behind you to clasp the hands and allow the torso to bend over the stretched out legs whilst stretching the arms up to the ceiling. Unclasp the hands and bring the arms to circle over the stretched out legs
    <u>Important note:</u>
    Take care on the circle of the arms when unclasping especially if you have weak shoulders
7. Roll back again bringing the legs overhead just as in the Roll Over exercise
8. Open and close the legs re crossing. This time your right ankle is crossed over the left ankle
9. Roll up into a V shape sitting position with legs stretched out in front of you at a 45-degree angle and arms stretched up by your ears
10. Lean forward till your legs touch the floor; take the arms in a circle behind you to clasp the hands and allow the torso to bend over the stretched out legs whilst stretching the arms up to the ceiling. Unclasp the hands and bring the arms to circle over the stretched out legs
11. Repeat this sequence 3 times

Benefits
The Boomerang allows for a complete body workout.

Watchfulness
Keep in mind that you always need to scoop the belly in towards the spine. Do not hold your breath; a continuous inhale on the peeling off the mat and exhale on the return of the spine towards the mat should be maintained throughout the exercise.

Do not do this exercise if you suffer from a slipped disk or you have a severe injured spine.

You have just completed The Boomerang exercise. Good work! Continue with The Rocking Chair when you feel comfortable to continue.

**Important Note: All Stockpiles should begin with Stockpile Workout 1
<u>Stockpile Workout 5</u>
The Crab
The Boomerang
Rocking Chair
The Can-Can
The Mermaids
Side Isometrics

The Rocking Chair
<u>Level 1—Technique</u>
1. Sit on your sitting bones at the edge of the mat
2. Bend your knees into your chest and open them to shoulder width. This will bring them in a 90-degree angle
3. Tilt back the torso to get balance and grasp under the thighs above the knees. Raise the feet so that the toes are slightly higher than knee height
4. Keep the elbows open looking to the sides; connect the shoulder blades and slide them down your spine
<u>Level 1—Workout</u>
5. Make that spine into a C-shape and begin to roll onto the mat vertebrae by vertebrae like a ball
6. Keep your head in and elbows out looking to the sides whilst you begin to roll onto the spine then roll back up again
7. Repeat sequence for 5 rolls
<u>Level 2—Technique</u>
8. Sit on your sitting bones at the edge of the mat
9. Straighten your legs, grasp the calves or ankles and open the legs shoulder width. This will bring them in a 90-degree angle
10. Tilt back the torso to get balance
11. Connect the shoulder blades and slide them down your spine to create a straight back line
<u>Level 2—Workout</u>
12. Make that spine into a C-shape and begin to roll onto the mat vertebrae by vertebrae like a ball
13. Keep your head in whilst you begin to roll onto the spine then roll back up again
14. When you have rolled up to the sitting level straighten that spine again
15. Repeat sequence for 5 rolls

Benefits
The Rocking Chair allows for a complete massage to the spinal column, stretches the hamstrings and stretches the entire back.

The abdominals (abdomen) are four abdominal muscles in partitions:
1. The Transverse Abdominal muscles are the deepest of the four that force the air from the lungs, hence the exhale acquired whilst lifting is initiated in abdominal exercises
2. The Rectus Abdominal muscle functions to flex the trunk. We can see this movement done when the body is in the C-shape spine position on the mat
3. Internal and External Obliques work to rotate the trunk

The hamstrings flex the knee and extend the thigh. The Rocking Chair exercise stretched the hamstrings, as too tight hamstrings can lead to spine problems. This can be noticed when one sits on the floor with legs stretched out in front.

Watchfulness
Keep in mind that you always need to scoop the belly in towards the spine when you initiate the roll to and from the mat. Do not hold your breath; a continuous inhale of rolling down and exhale of rolling up should be maintained throughout the exercise.

Try to keep your shoulders pressed away from your ears in order to eliminate the shrugging of shoulders. Stop the roll of the spine at the shoulder blades and never onto the neck area.

You have just completed The Rocking Chair exercise. Good work! Continue with The Can-Can when you feel comfortable to continue.

**Important Note: All Stockpiles should begin with Stockpile Workout 1
<u>Stockpile Workout 5</u>
The Crab
The Boomerang
Rocking Chair
The Can-Can
The Mermaids
Side Isometrics

The Can-Can

<u>Technique</u>
1.   Sit up on your mat and take those arms behind you for support. If you have a delicate lower back, rest upon the elbows
2.   Turn the hip to the right then stretch the legs diagonally in a Pilates Stance. This will bring the legs to a diagonal 45-degree angle (Fig. 1)
<u>Workout</u>
3.   Begin to draw 6 small circles in the air with your toes
4.   When the circles are drawn, bend the legs and change side
<u>Technique</u>
5.   Turn the hip to the left then stretch the legs diagonally in a Pilates Stance. This will bring the legs to a diagonal 45-degree angle
<u>Workout</u>
6.   Begin to draw 6 small circles in the air with your toes to repeat for 6 small circles on the other side
7.   When the circles are drawn, bend the legs and change side
<u>Technique</u>
8.   Turn the hip to the right then stretch the legs diagonally in a Pilates Stance but now flex the feet. This will bring the legs to a diagonal 45-degree angle in a Charlie Chaplin Stance
<u>Workout</u>
9.   Begin to draw 6 small circles in the air with your heels
10.   When the circles are drawn, bend the legs and change side
<u>Technique</u>
11.   Turn the hip to the left then stretch the legs diagonally in a Pilates Stance but now flex the feet. This will bring the legs to a diagonal 45-degree angle in a Charlie Chaplin Stance
<u>Workout</u>
12.   Begin to draw 6 small circles in the air with your heels
13.   When the circles are drawn, bend the legs and rest

<u>Benefits</u>
The Can-Can is a complete body workout, initiates the arms, chest, shoulders and abdominal area.

The abdominals (abdomen) are four abdominal muscles in partitions:
1. The Transverse Abdominal muscles are the deepest of the four that force the air from the lungs, hence the exhale acquired whilst lifting is initiated in abdominal exercises
2. The Rectus Abdominal muscle functions to flex the trunk. We can see this movement done when the body is in the C-shape spine position on the mat
3. Internal and External Obliques work to rotate the trunk

<u>Watchfulness</u>
Do not hold your breath; a continuous inhale of 3 circles and exhale of 3 circles should be maintained throughout the exercise.

Try to keep your shoulders pressed away from your ears in order to eliminate the shrugging of shoulders. Should you feel uncomfortable with your arms supporting you, rest the weight of your body onto your elbows (Fig.1).

You have just completed The Can-Can exercise. Good work! Continue with The Mermaids when you feel comfortable to continue.

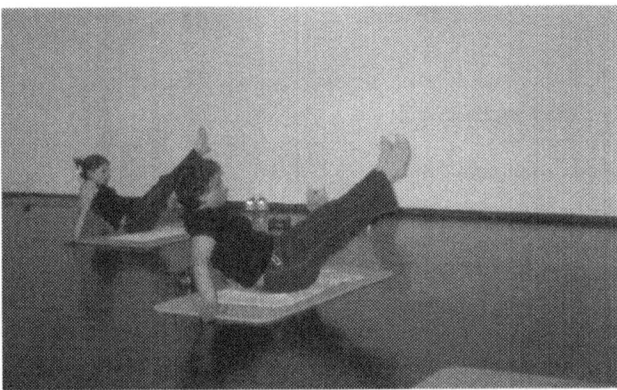

Fig. 1

**Important Note: All Stockpiles should begin with Stockpile Workout 1

<u>Stockpile Workout 5</u>

The Crab

The Boomerang

Rocking Chair

The Can-Can

The Mermaids

Side Isometrics

The Mermaids

<u>Technique—Level 1</u>

1. Sit on your right hip side. Bend those legs and take them to the left side of your body. This will bring the legs to a 90-degree angle

2. Grasp your left ankle with your left hand for support and take your right hand to stretch towards the ceiling next to your ear. Try to lower the shoulder from the ear to avoid the shrugging motion

3. Straighten the spine by connecting the shoulder blades together and sliding them down your spine. Imagine you are sitting against an imaginary wall for support

   <u>Workout—Level 1</u>

4. Bend your torso to the left side towards the ankles and feel the stretch on your right side. You are now in the Mermaid position (Fig. 1)

5. Hold this position for 5 inhales and 5 exhales

6. Come back to neutral position. Repeat 3 times before changing sides

   <u>Technique—Level 2</u>

7. Come back to your Mermaid position (Fig. 1)

   <u>Workout—Level 2</u>

8. Bring your right palm to the floor and rest the elbow on the mat

9. As you are in that curve, stretch your left arm towards the ceiling in a diagonal movement next to your left ear

10. Come back to the Mermaid position and repeat this sequence 3 times to each side

    <u>Technique—Level 3</u>

11. Come back to your Mermaid position (Fig. 1)

    <u>Workout—Level 3</u>

12. Take your right arm and stretch it onto the mat so your upper body is lying on its side and your head is resting on your right arm

13. Now stretch your left arm towards the ceiling in a diagonal movement next to your left ear

14. Push up on your right arm to come back to the Mermaid position (Fig. 1)

15. Repeat this sequence 3 times on each side

Benefits
The Mermaid initiates the waistline.

Watchfulness
Do not hold your breath; a continuous inhale of 5 and exhale of 5 should be maintained throughout the exercise.

Try to keep your shoulders pressed away from your ears in order to eliminate the shrugging of shoulders. Always imagine your spine is supported against an imaginary wall whilst in the Mermaid position. (Fig. 1)

You have just completed The Mermaids exercise. Good work! Continue with the Side Isometrics when you feel comfortable to continue.

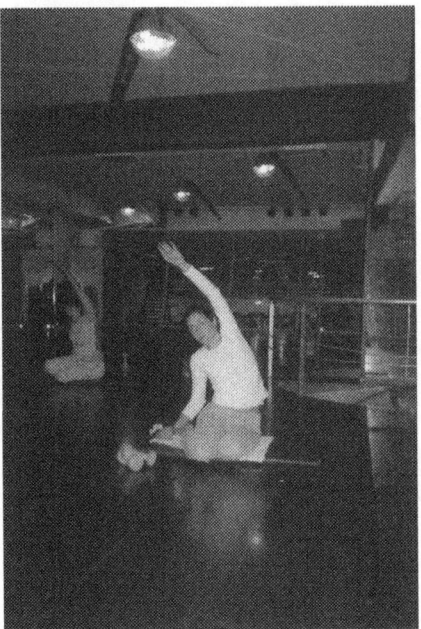

Fig. 1

**Important Note: All Stockpiles should begin with Stockpile Workout 1

<u>Stockpile Workout 5</u>
The Crab
The Boomerang
Rocking Chair
The Can-Can
The Mermaids
Side Isometrics

Side Isometrics

<u>Technique—Level 1</u>

1. Sit onto your right hip and bring your right palm to the floor. Have the palm placed under the shoulder line

   <u>Important note:</u>

   To protect the wrist, put most of the body weight onto the beginning of the palm and not on the center of the palm or on the inside of the knuckles

   <u>Workout—Level 1</u>

2. Come on up on your right knee and have it placed in line with the hip joint (Fig. 1)

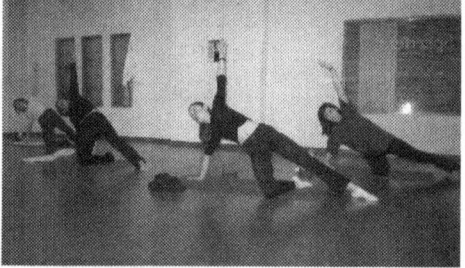

Fig. 1

3. Bring your left arm to stretch to the ceiling with palm facing forward. Try to get both arms to form one straight line. Look up at your palm for 5 counts and then slowly bring your right hip to rest once again on the mat. Repeat 3 times to each side

   <u>Technique—Level 2</u>

4. Sit onto your right hip and bring your right palm to the floor. Have the palm placed under the shoulder line

   <u>Workout—Level 2</u>

5. Come onto your right knee and place it in line with the hip joint (Fig. 1).

6. Stretch your left arm to the ceiling with palm facing forward. Try to get both arms to form one straight line. Take the bent leg and stretch it behind the left (Fig. 2)

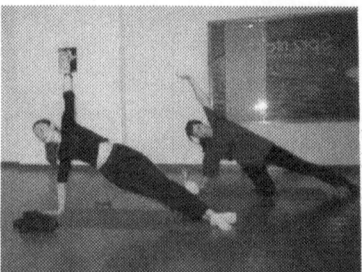

Fig. 2

7. Look up at your palm for 5 counts and then bring your right knee to rest once again on the mat (Fig. 1) then slowly bring your right hip down. Repeat 3 times each side
Technique—Level 3

8. Sit onto your right hip, bring the right palm to the floor and place it under the shoulder. Bend your right leg and cross your left leg over the right ankle (Fig. 3)

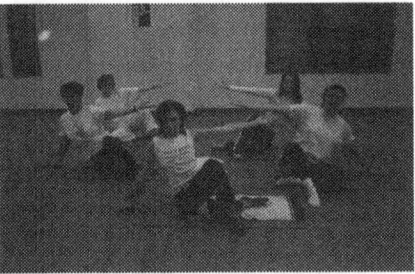

Fig. 3

9. Take your left hand to stretch out beside you with palm facing up
Workout—Level 3

10. Lift your hips off the mat, straighten both legs and twist the hips towards the ceiling allowing you to take the left hand under your torso for that twist—imagine your torso is a bridge and you want to pass under it (Fig. 4)

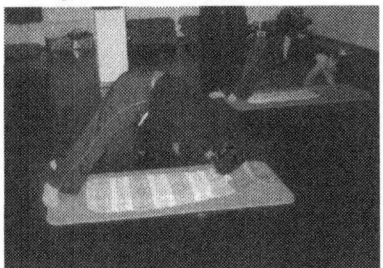

Fig. 4

11. Keep your head tucked in as it follows the left arm under the bridge. Hold this position for 3 counts and then slowly bring your entire body, hips first, to rest once again on the mat. Repeat this movement 3 times each side

Benefits

The Side Isometrics initiate the whole body, strengthens the shoulder and wrist. When great force is initiated on the shoulder, it is vital that the scapula (shoulder blade) is fixed in place and kept against the ribcage.

Watchfulness

Do not hold your breath; a continuous inhale of 5 and exhale of 5 should be maintained throughout the exercise. Try not to demolish onto the shoulder that is being used to eliminate any additional tension. Remember, do levels 2 & 3 only when you are familiar with the basic level and your shoulder has strengthened.

You have just completed The Side Isometrics exercise and Stockpile 5. Good work!

IMPROVEMENT RECORD STOCKPILE WORKOUT 5

The Crab

The Boomerang

Rocking Chair

IMPROVEMENT RECORD STOCKPILE WORKOUT 5

The Can-Can

The Mermaids

Side Isometrics

**Important Note: All Stockpiles should begin with Stockpile Workout 1

<u>Stockpile Workout 6</u>
Side Lifts
All Leg Side Lifts
Inner Thigh Lifts
Inside Leg Circle
Archer's Legs

Side Lifts

<u>Technique—Level 1</u>

1. Lie onto your right side and stretch out with your head resting upon your right arm
2. Bring the left arm to rest onto your left hip with palm facing down. Bring those legs in a Pilates Stance and zip up the inner thighs
   <u>Workout—Level 1</u>
3. Raise both legs to the level that your hip flexibility will allow, and then lower to the mat without touching the floor. Repeat this 3 times
4. After you have done the repetitions, you will now add the torso to lift together with your legs. Imagine ribs and legs want to meet to diminish that gap between the rib bones and pelvis. Repeat this 3 times and change sides
5. When you are accustomed to this basic level go onto level 2
   <u>Technique—Level 2</u>
6. Lie onto your right side and stretch out with your head resting upon your right arm and fingertips pointing on the mat. Keep the left arm diagonally in front of you
7. Bring those legs in a Pilates Stance with zipped up inner thighs diagonally before you (Fig. 1). This will bring the legs to a 45-degree angle
   <u>Workout—Level 2</u>
8. Raise both legs up to the level that your hip flexibility will allow, together with your torso. The fingertips help push up your body weight
9. Repeat 5 times before lowering to the mat. Change sides
   <u>Technique—Level 3</u>
10. Lie onto your right side and stretch out with your head resting upon your right arm and fingertips pointing on the mat. Keep the left arm diagonally in front of you
11. Bring those legs in a Pilates Stance with zipped up inner thighs diagonally before you (Fig. 1). This will bring the legs to a 45-degree angle
    <u>Workout—Level 3</u>
12. Tilt back your pelvis to almost sit onto the side of your hip, raise the legs and torso simultaneously with fingertips helping you push up (Fig. 2)
13. Pulse the legs for 2 counts and bring them back down
14. Repeat 5 times before lowering to the mat

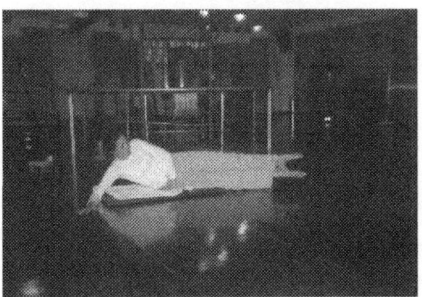

Fig. 1

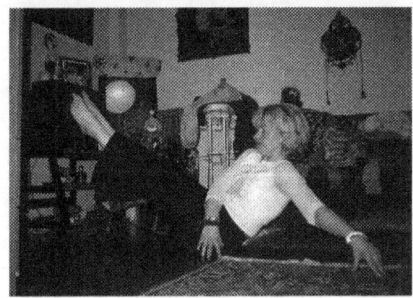

Fig. 2

<u>Benefits</u>
The Side Lifts are complete body workouts.

<u>Watchfulness</u>
Do not hold your breath; a continuous inhale of 5 and exhale of 5 should be maintained throughout the exercise.

Try not to demolish onto the shoulder that is being used to hold you up to eliminate any additional tension. Remember, do levels 2 & 3 only when you are familiar with the basic level and your body has strengthened enough.

You have just completed The Side Lifts. Good work! Continue with All Side Leg Lift Series when you feel comfortable to continue.

**Important Note: All Stockpiles should begin with Stockpile Workout 1

Stockpile Workout 6

Side Lifts

All Side Leg Lift Series

   Hot potato

   Single Side Leg Circle

   Side Kick

   Seated Leg Lift

   The Oyster

Inner Thigh Lifts

Inside Leg Circle

Archer's Legs

Hot Potato

Technique

1. Lie onto your right side and stretch out with your palm supporting your head
2. Keep the left arm diagonally in front of you
3. Form the Pilates Stance and zip up the inner thighs

Workout

4. Keep your right leg on the floor; take the top leg to cross over and pulse for 3 small beats with toes touching the floor. Take the leg back and pulse to the back for 3 small beats with toes touching the floor
5. Repeat these alternating small pulses 10 times before changing sides

Benefits
The Hot Potato initiates the entire leg.

Watchfulness
Do not hold your breath; a continuous natural inhale and exhale should be maintained throughout the exercise.

Try not to demolish onto the shoulder whilst resting your head on your palm to eliminate any additional tension.

You have just completed The Hot Potato. Good work! Continue with the Single Side Leg Circle from this series when you feel comfortable to continue.

**Important Note: All Stockpiles should begin with Stockpile Workout 1

<u>Stockpile Workout 6</u>

Side Lifts

All Side Leg Lift Series

> Hot potato
>
> Single Side Leg Circle
>
> Side Kick
>
> Seated Leg Lift
>
> The Oyster

Inner Thigh Lifts

Inside Leg Circle

Archer's Legs

Single Side Leg Circle

<u>Technique</u>

1. Lie onto your right side and stretch out with your palm supporting your head
2. Keep the left arm diagonally in front of you with your palm on the mat for support
3. Take those legs into a Pilates Stance and zip up the inner thighs

<u>Workout</u>

4. Keep your right leg on the floor and with your left leg begin to draw 10 small circles one way, then 10 small circles the other way before changing sides
5. Keep the range of motion small and try to work the leg in line with your hip

Benefits
The Single Side Leg Circle initiates the entire leg and adds strength to the hip joint.

When the pelvis moves forward at the hip joint (anterior superior iliac spine), it increases Lordosis (inward curve of the lower back).

Watchfulness
Do not hold your breath; a continuous natural inhale and exhale should be maintained throughout the exercise.

Try to keep the whole body stable without rocking the pelvis as you draw the circles with your leg to acquire the benefits of this exercise.

You have just completed The Single Side Leg Circle. Good work! Continue with the Side Kick from this series when you feel comfortable to continue.

**Important Note: All Stockpiles should begin with Stockpile Workout 1

<u>Stockpile Workout 6</u>
Side Lifts
All Side Leg Lift Series
    Hot potato
    Single Side Leg Circle
    Side Kick
    Seated Leg Lift
    The Oyster
Inner Thigh Lifts
Inside Leg Circle
Archer's Legs

Side Kick

<u>Technique—Level 1</u>

1. Lie onto your right side and stretch out with your palm supporting your head
2. Keep the left arm diagonally in front of you with your palm on the mat for support
3. Take those legs in a Pilates Stance and zip up the inner thighs
4. Keep your right leg on the floor with toes pressed into the mat for stabilization of the whole body

<u>Workout—Level 1</u>

5. Take your left leg flexed and begin to kick forward in front of you as far as you can. On bringing the leg back, point the toes
6. Repeat 5 kicks before changing sides

<u>Technique—Level 2</u>

7. Sit up onto your right hip and bring your right palm to the floor. Have the palm placed under the shoulder line

<u>Important note:</u>

To protect the wrist, put most of the body weight onto the beginning of the palm and not on the center of the palm or on the inside of the knuckles

8. Come on up on your right knee and have it placed in line with the hip joint
9. Bring your left palm to the back of your head or keep it on the side of your hip

<u>Workout—Level 2</u>

10. Raise your left leg flexed in one line with your torso and begin to kick forward in front of you as far as you can. On bringing the leg back, point the toes
11. Repeat 5 kicks before changing sides Do not lower that leg till the exercise is finished

Benefits

The Side Leg Kick initiates the inner thighs (adductors) and outer thighs (abductors), and adds strength to the hip joint. The major action in abduction of the leg is done by the Gluteus Medius.

When the pelvis moves forward at the hip joint (anterior superior iliac spine), it increases Lordosis (inward curve of the lower back).

Watchfulness

Do not hold your breath; a continuous natural inhale and exhale should be maintained throughout the exercise.

Try to keep the whole body stable without rocking as you kick forward and don't work lower than your bodyline to acquire the benefits of this exercise.

You have just completed The Side Leg Kick. Good work! Continue with the Seated Leg Lift from this series when you feel comfortable to continue.

**Important Note: All Stockpiles should begin with Stockpile Workout 1

<u>Stockpile Workout 6</u>

Side Lifts

All Side Leg Lift Series

       Hot potato

       Single Side Leg Circle

       Side Kick

       Seated Leg Lift

       The Oyster

Inner Thigh Lifts

Inside Leg Circle

Archer's Legs

Seated Leg Lift

<u>Technique</u>

1. Sit on your left hip and bend those legs keeping the left leg in front of you and take the right leg passed your hip behind the pelvis
2. Rest both palms in front of you for support

<u>Workout</u>

3. Raise that back leg that is still bent for 5 counts then keep it up and begin to pulse it for another 5 counts (Fig. 1)
4. Change sides

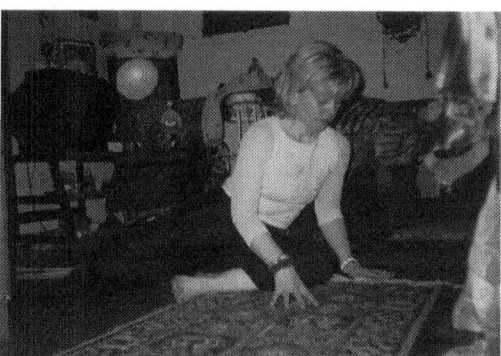

Fig. 1

Benefits

The Seated Leg Lift initiates the entire leg particularly targeting the buttocks.

When the knee is in a lateral rotation as in the Seated Leg Lift, the following muscles are initiated.

1. Tensor Fasciae Latae that often becomes hypertonic (over tense)
2. Gluteus Maximus that can be the cause for lower back problems due to Lordosis
3. Biceps Femoris on the outside of the thigh

Watchfulness

Do not hold your breath; a continuous natural inhale and exhale should be maintained throughout the exercise.

Try to keep the whole body stable without rocking backwards and forwards as you raise that back leg. In time, your body will get used to this awkward position and be more comfortable.

You have just completed The Seated Leg Lift. Good work! Continue with The Oyster from this series when you feel comfortable to continue.

**Important Note: All Stockpiles should begin with Stockpile Workout 1
<u>Stockpile Workout 6</u>
Side Lifts
All Side Leg Lift Series
       Hot potato
       Single Side Leg Circle
       Side Kick
       Seated Leg Lift
       The Oyster
Inner Thigh Lifts
Inside Leg Circle
Archer's Legs

The Oyster

<u>Technique</u>

1. Lie on your right side resting your head on your palm for support
2. Bend both legs and bring them in front of you with knees looking forward. This will bring the legs to a 90-degree angle
3. Bring those legs to a downward turn so the knees are now facing the mat
4. Keep the insides of your feet glued together

<u>Workout</u>

5. Raise the top leg as wide as it feels comfortable (Fig.1) then bring it back to its original position—imagine the top leg is the top cap of an oyster as it opens and closes
6. Repeat this sequence 10 times then keep the top leg open and begin to pulse it for 10 counts before changing sides

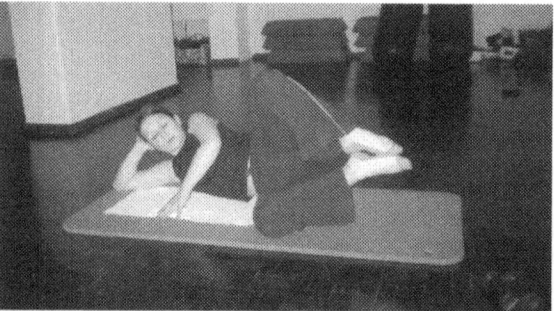

Fig. 1

Benefits
The Oyster initiates the entire leg particularly targeting the hips and buttocks.

When the knee is in a lateral rotation as in the Seated Leg Lift, the following muscles are initiated.
1. Tensor Fasciae Latae that often becomes hypertonic (over tense)
2. Gluteus Maximus that can be the cause for lower back problems due to Lordosis
3. Biceps Femoris on the outside of the thigh

Watchfulness
Do not hold your breath; a continuous natural inhale and exhale should be maintained throughout the exercise.

Try to keep the whole body stable without rocking backwards and forwards as you open and close the top leg. Try not to demolish onto the palm as it holds your head weight to eliminate any additional tension.

You have just completed The Oyster. Good work! Continue with the Inner Thigh Lifts when you feel comfortable to continue.

**Important Note: All Stockpiles should begin with Stockpile Workout 1
<u>Stockpile Workout 6</u>
Side Lifts
All Side Leg Lift Series
       Hot potato
       Single Side Leg Circle
       Side Kick
       Seated Leg Lift
       The Oyster
Inner Thigh Lifts
Inside Leg Circle
Archer's Legs

Inner Thigh Lifts

<u>Technique</u>
1.   Lie stretched out onto your right side with your palm supporting your head
2.   Bend the left leg and cross it over the right leg so the left sole is on the mat in front of the right leg
3.   Flex the right foot and do an outward turn of the thigh so that the toes are looking down
    <u>Workout</u>
4.   Raise that bottom leg for 10 counts as high as it will go then keep the bottom leg up and begin to pulse it for 10 counts before changing sides

Benefits
The Inner Thigh Lifts initiates and tones the inner thighs (adductors).

Watchfulness
Do not hold your breath; a continuous natural inhale and exhale should be maintained throughout the exercise.

Try to keep the bottom foot flexed and turned towards the mat to establish a quality effect. Try not to demolish onto the palm as it holds your head weight to eliminate any additional tension.

You have just completed the Inner Thigh Lifts. Good work! Continue with the Inside Leg Circle when you feel comfortable to continue.

**Important Note: All Stockpiles should begin with Stockpile Workout 1
<u>Stockpile Workout 6</u>
Side Lifts
All Side Leg Lift Series
   Hot potato
   Single Side Leg Circle
   Side Kick
   Seated Leg Lift
   The Oyster
Inner Thigh Lifts
Inside Leg Circle
Archer's Legs

Inside Leg Circle

<u>Technique</u>

1. Lie stretched out onto your right side with your palm supporting your head
2. Bend the left leg and cross it over the right leg so the left sole is on the mat in front of the right leg
3. Flex the right foot and do an outward turn at the thigh so that the toes are looking down

<u>Workout</u>

4. Raise that bottom leg and draw 10 small circles in the air one way with the heel, then 10 small circles the other way with the heel before changing sides

Benefits
The Inside Leg Circle initiates and tones the inner thighs (adductors).

Watchfulness
Do not hold your breath; a continuous natural inhale and exhale should be maintained throughout the exercise.

Try to keep the bottom foot flexed and turned towards the mat as you draw those circles in the air to establish a quality effect. Try not to demolish onto the palm as it holds your head weight to eliminate any additional tension.

You have just completed the Inside Leg Circle. Good work! Continue with the Archer's Legs when you feel comfortable to continue.

**Important Note: All Stockpiles should begin with Stockpile Workout 1
<u>Stockpile Workout 6</u>
Side Lifts
All Side Leg Lift Series
      Hot potato
      Single Side Leg Circle
      Side Kick
      Seated Leg Lift
      The Oyster
Inner Thigh Lifts
Inside Leg Circle
Archer's Legs

Archer's Legs
<u>Technique</u>
1. Lie stretched out onto your left side with your head supported by your palm
2. Bend the right leg and have your toes gently touch the inside of the left leg
3. Point the left foot and do an outward turn from the hip joint so that the toes are looking down (Fig. 1)

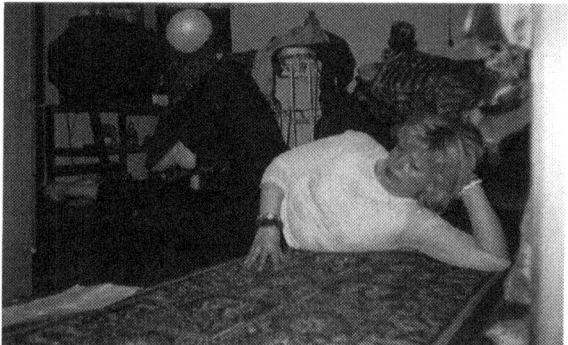

Fig.1

<u>Workout</u>
4. Straighten and bend the top leg 10 times
5. Now keep the toes touching the inside of the left leg, and raise and lower both legs simultaneously off the floor for 10 counts before you change sides

Benefits
The Archer's Legs initiates the entire leg and also tones the Sartorius muscle.

The Sartorius muscle abducts the hip, flexes the knee, and if it is hypertonic (over-tense) it can initiate stress on the inside of the knee.

Watchfulness
Do not hold your breath; a continuous natural inhale and exhale should be maintained throughout the exercise.

Try to keep the bottom foot turned towards the mat from the thigh. Try not to demolish onto the palm as it holds your head weight to eliminate any additional tension.

You have just completed the Archer's Leg and Stockpile 6. Good work!

IMPROVEMENT RECORD STOCKPILE WORKOUT 6

Side Lifts

All Side Leg Lift Series
    Hot potato

    Single Side Leg Circle

    Side Kick

    Seated Leg Lift

    The Oyster

IMPROVEMENT RECORD STOCKPILE WORKOUT 6

Inner Thigh Lifts

Inside Leg Circle

Archer's Legs

**Important Note: All Stockpiles should begin with Stockpile Workout 1

Stockpile Workout 7

The Ballerinas

The Ballerinas

Technique—Ballerina One

1. Sit cross-legged. Imagine your spine is supported against a wall. Bend those arms so that the elbows are looking out to the sides and palms facing your chest (Fig. 1). This will bring the elbow to a 45-degree angle

Workout—Ballerina One

2. Take the arms back to connect the shoulder blades (adduction) and your elbows are looking at the back wall. Slide those arms down your side and feel the shoulder blades slide down (depress). The elbows are now looking to the mat. Raise the bent arms over your head with palms looking down at the top of your head. To end the Ballerina One, bring the arms back to their original position and repeat 2 more times

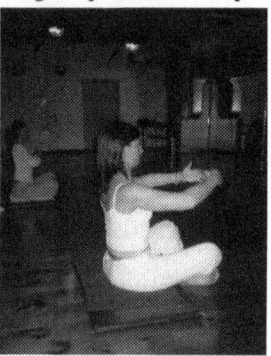

Fig. 1

Technique—Ballerina Two

3. Sit cross-legged and take your right leg to stretch out to the side with pointed toes. This brings the leg to do a diagonal 45-degree angle. Keep the left leg bent, and imagine your spine is resting against a wall. Bend those arms so that the elbows are looking out to the sides and raise the arms above your head with palms now facing the top of your head.

Workout—Ballerina Two

4. Twist your torso towards the bent leg (left leg here). Keep the elbows open and looking to the sides. Bend your torso towards your extended leg (right leg here). If your right elbow does not touch the leg don't worry about it. Flexibility will improve. (Fig. 2). Raise the torso to its twist to the left then come back to the original position. Repeat 2 more times

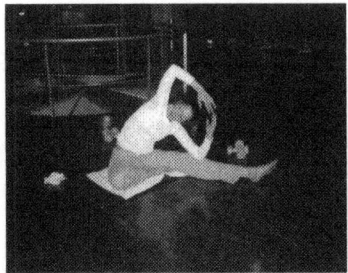

Fig. 2

<u>Technique—Ballerina Three</u>

5. Remain seated and take your right flexed leg to stretch forward out in front of you. This will bring the leg to a 90-degree angle. Keep the left leg bent closely to you. Imagine your spine is supported against a wall. Take those arms and stretch them up towards the ceiling. Bend at the elbows and take those fingertips to your upper back

<u>Workout—Ballerina Three</u>

6. Walk those fingertips as far down your back as you can, keeping the elbows out and looking towards the ceiling (Fig. 3). With this aligned spine, bend your torso forward and hold this position for 10 counts before changing legs to repeat the exercise

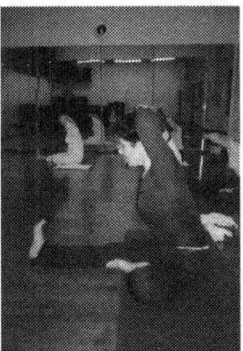

Fig. 3

<u>Benefits</u>

The Ballerinas initiates the whole back, reduces Lordosis (the in curve of the lower back) and Kyphosis (hunched and rolled in shoulders). All Ballerina exercises initiate the scapula (shoulder blade).

<u>Watchfulness</u>

Do not hold your breath; a continuous natural inhale and exhale should be maintained throughout the exercise. If you notice that you are too uncomfortable in the Ballerinas position, sit on a folded towel to bring the height of your hips above your knee level

Always imagine a wall where your entire spine is supported against it. Try not to actually rest against a wall in order to get the benefits of these exercises.

You have just completed the Ballerinas and Stockpile 7. Good work!

IMPROVEMENT RECORD STOCKPILE WORKOUT 7

The Ballerinas

IMPROVEMENT RECORD STOCKPILE WORKOUT 7

The Ballerinas

**Important Note: All Stockpiles should begin with Stockpile Workout 1

<u>Stockpile Workout 8</u>

Butt Chopper

The Pigeon (Yoga Asana)

Butt Chopper

<u>Technique—Level 1</u>

1. Lie on your stomach with legs shoulder distance apart and have your forehead rest on the back of your hands

2. Have the legs in a Pilates Stance before rising in the air to shoulder width. Squeeze the buttocks (Fig. 1)

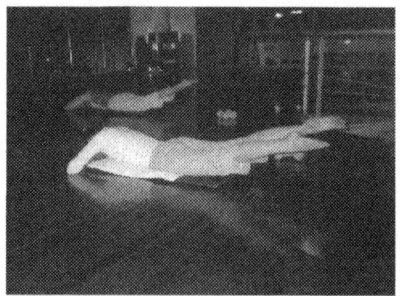

Fig. 1

<u>Workout—Level 1</u>

3. Open the legs wider, close the legs and bend the knees to bring the heels towards your buttocks (Fig. 2)

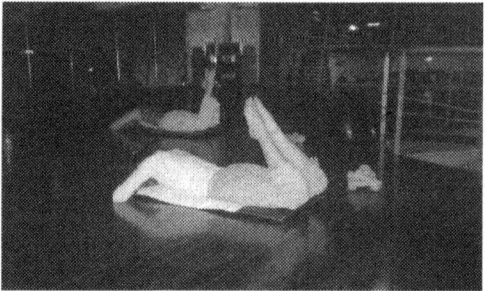

Fig. 2

4. Straighten your legs again to repeat the sequence

<u>Important note:</u>

Do Level 1 about 4-5 times or as many times as you feel comfortable. Keep the legs off the floor whilst doing the exercise and keep squeezing the buttocks to help keep those legs up against gravity. If you feel any tension in your lower back, lower the legs slightly to the floor, but try not to let the knee touch the mat

<u>Technique—Level 2</u>

5. Lie on your stomach with legs shoulder distance apart and palms at your side facing the floor. Bend the legs keeping the inside of the soles glued together (Fig. 3)

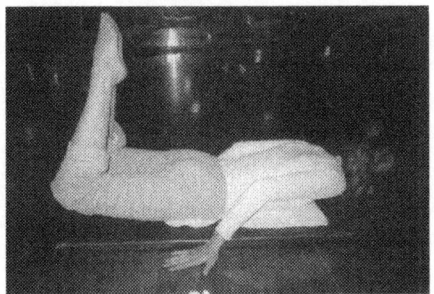

Fig. 3

<u>Workout—Level 2</u>

6. Raise the legs straight up to the ceiling. This will take them to a 90-degree angle. Squeeze the buttocks to help those legs up against gravity and have the palms press into the floor to help. Lower the legs and repeat the sequence 5 more times

7. When you have completed 5 raises, keep the legs up and slowly open and close the knees for 5 counts or as many times you feel comfortable. Try not to unglue the feet; always keep them together

<u>Benefits</u>

The Butt Chopper tones and firms the buttocks.

<u>Watchfulness</u>

Do not hold your breath; a continuous natural inhale and exhale should be maintained throughout the exercise.

You have just completed the Butt Chopper. Good work! Continue with The Pigeon (Yoga Asana) when you feel comfortable to continue.

**Important Note: All Stockpiles should begin with Stockpile Workout 1

<u>Stockpile Workout 8</u>

Butt Chopper

The Pigeon (Yoga Asana)

The Pigeon (Yoga Asana)

<u>Technique</u>

1. Come onto your hands and knees in cat position

<u>Workout</u>

2. Slide your right knee forward between the hands. Slide the left leg back as you lower your hips to the mat
3. Press your palms into the mat for support and reach the crown of the head up
4. Lean forward to rest the chest onto the right leg stretching the hands forward
5. Remain for 3-6 breaths before changing sides

Benefits
The Pigeon initiates the Piriformis muscle that does not allow you to do the splits. This muscle rotates the thigh laterally (turns it out) and is very weak becoming hypertonic (over-tense).

Watchfulness
Do not hold your breath; a continuous natural inhale and exhale should be maintained throughout the exercise.

You have just completed The Pigeon and Stockpile 8. Good work!

IMPROVEMENT RECORD STOCKPILE WORKOUT 8

Butt Chopper

IMPROVEMENT RECORD STOCKPILE WORKOUT 8

The Pigeon (Yoga Asana)

**Important Note: All Stockpiles should begin with Stockpile Workout 1
<u>Stockpile Workout 9</u>
The Seal
Rowing
Spine Twists
The Saw
Russian Curl
Spine Stretch Forward

The Seal
<u>Technique</u>
1.   Sit on the edge of your mat with your legs bent to the chest and pass the hands under and inside so that your palms are resting against the outside of your ankles
2.   Tilt back slightly to balance on your sit bones (*See Pictures from The Crab exercise*)
<u>Workout</u>
3.   Keep your head tucked in, clap the soles of your feet together 3 times then begin to roll onto the spine vertebrae by vertebrae like a ball
<u>Important note:</u>
Stop the roll of the spine at the shoulder blades and never onto the neck area
4.   Clap the soles 3 times again then roll back up to the original position
5.   Repeat 5 times

Benefits

The Seal allows for a complete massage to the spinal column.

Watchfulness

Keep in mind that you always need to scoop the belly in towards the spine. Do not hold your breath; a continuous inhale of rolling down and exhale of rolling up should be maintained throughout the exercise.

Try to keep your shoulders pressed away from your ears in order to eliminate the shrugging of shoulders. Stop the roll of the spine at the shoulder blades and never onto the neck area.

You have just completed The Seal exercise. Good work! Continue with the Rowing when you feel comfortable to continue.

**Important Note: All Stockpiles should begin with Stockpile Workout 1

<u>Stockpile Workout 9</u>

The Seal

Rowing

Spine Twists

The Saw

Russian Curl

Spine Stretch Forward

Rowing

<u>Technique</u>

1. Sit on the edge of your mat with your legs stretched out in front of you in a Pilates Stance and zip up the inner thighs

2. Bend the elbows to your side so the elbows are looking behind you with palms facing the floor. Imagine your spine is resting against an imaginary wall

<u>Important note:</u>

If you feel too uncomfortable in this position, sit on a folded towel to bring the height of your hips above your knee level

<u>Workout</u>

3. Stretch the arms in front of you, lower them towards your legs, take them up positioning them next to your ears, and then take them wide out to the side with palms facing the back wall before your begin from initial position again

4. Repeat the sequence 3-5 times

5. Weights of 1kg (2.2 lb) can be used to add extra intensity

Benefits
The Rowing initiates spinal alignment and works the shoulder in its socket.

Watchfulness
Do not hold your breath; a continuous inhale and exhale should be maintained throughout the exercise.

Try to keep your shoulders pressed away from your ears in order to eliminate the shrugging of shoulders.

You have just completed the Rowing. Good work! Continue with the Spine Twists when you feel comfortable to continue.

**Important Note: All Stockpiles should begin with Stockpile Workout 1

<u>Stockpile Workout 9</u>

The Seal

Rowing

Spine Twists

The Saw

Russian Curl

Spine Stretch Forward

Spine Twists

<u>Technique—Level 1</u>

1. Sit on the edge of your mat with your legs flexed out in front of you at shoulder width distance

2. Bring your arms out to your sides in a straight line with your shoulders so that your palms are facing the floor. Imagine your spine is resting against an imaginary wall (Fig. 1)

    <u>Important note:</u>

    If you feel too uncomfortable in this position, sit on a folded towel to bring the height of your hips above your knee level

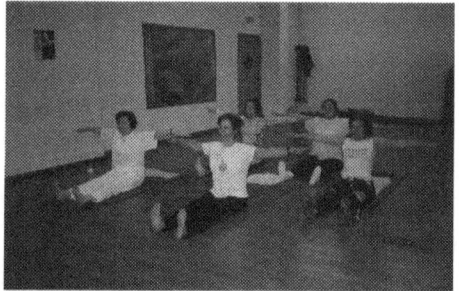

Fig. 1

<u>Workout—Level 1</u>

3. Begin to twist the torso to the right without moving the hips or legs. Ground the pelvis to the mat. Inhale

4. Twist the torso back to original position (Fig. 1). Exhale

5. Repeat the sequence 3 times to each side

    <u>Technique—Level 2</u>

6. Sit on the edge of your mat with your legs flexed out in front of you at shoulder width distance

7. Bring your arms out to your sides in a straight line with your shoulders so that your palms are facing the floor. Imagine your spine is resting against an imaginary wall (Fig. 1)

    <u>Important note:</u>

    If you feel too uncomfortable in this position, sit on a folded towel to bring the height of your hips above your knee level

Workout—Level 2

8. Twist the torso to the right and pulse for 3 counts without moving the hips or legs. Ground the pelvis to the mat
9. Twist the torso back to original position, bend the legs towards you sliding the heels on the floor then straighten again before changing sides
10. Repeat this sequence 3 times to each side

Benefits

The Spine Twists initiates spinal alignment, aims to help with Scoliosis, works the shoulder in its socket, and initiates the oblique abdominal area.

The abdominals (abdomen) are four abdominal muscles in partitions:

1. The Transverse Abdominal muscles are the deepest of the four that force the air from the lungs, hence the exhale acquired whilst lifting is initiated in abdominal exercises
2. The Rectus Abdominal muscle functions to flex the trunk. We can see this movement done when the body is in the C-shape spine position on the mat
3. Internal and External Obliques work to rotate the trunk

Watchfulness

Do not hold your breath; a continuous inhale and exhale should be maintained throughout the exercise. Try to keep your shoulders pressed away from your ears in order to eliminate the shrugging of shoulders.

You have just completed The Spine Twists exercise. Good work! Continue with The Saw when you feel comfortable to continue.

**Important Note: All Stockpiles should begin with Stockpile Workout 1
<u>Stockpile Workout 9</u>
The Seal
Rowing
Spine Twists
The Saw
Russian Curl
Spine Stretch Forward

The Saw

<u>Technique</u>
1. Sit on the edge of your mat with your legs flexed out in front of you at shoulder width distance
2. Bring your arms out to your sides in a straight line with your shoulders so that your palms are facing the floor. Imagine your spine is resting against an imaginary wall *(See Fig. 1 from Spine Twists exercise)*
    <u>Important note:</u>
    If you feel too uncomfortable in this position, sit on a folded towel to bring the height of your hips above your knee level
    <u>Workout</u>
3. Begin to twist the torso to the right without moving the hips or legs. Ground the pelvis to the mat
4. Bend forward so that the left hand passes the outside of the right flexed foot (Fig. 1)
5. Raise into the sitting position again and twist the torso back to original position before changing sides
6. Repeat this sequence 3 times to each side

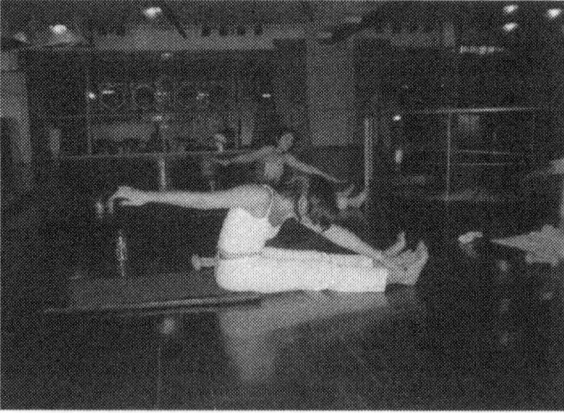

Fig. 1

Benefits
The Saw initiates spinal alignment, works the shoulder in its socket, aims to help in Scoliosis, and initiates the oblique abdominal area.

The abdominals (abdomen) are four abdominal muscles in partitions:
1. The Transverse Abdominal muscles are the deepest of the four that force the air from the lungs, hence the exhale acquired whilst lifting is initiated in abdominal exercises
2. The Rectus Abdominal muscle functions to flex the trunk. We can see this movement done when the body is in the C-shape spine position on the mat
3. Internal and External Obliques work to rotate the trunk

Watchfulness
Do not hold your breath; a continuous inhale and exhale should be maintained throughout the exercise. Try to keep your shoulders pressed away from your ears in order to eliminate the shrugging of shoulders.

You have just completed The Saw exercise. Good work! Continue with the Russian Curl when you feel comfortable to continue.

**Important Note: All Stockpiles should begin with Stockpile Workout 1
<u>Stockpile Workout 9</u>
The Seal
Rowing
Spine Twists
The Saw
Russian Curl
Spine Stretch Forward

Russian Curl

1. Sit on the edge of your mat with your legs in a Pilates Stance with pointed toes
2. Fold your arms in front of your chest
3. Scoop the torso into a C-shape spine and tilt back squeezing the front thighs for extra support (Fig. 1)

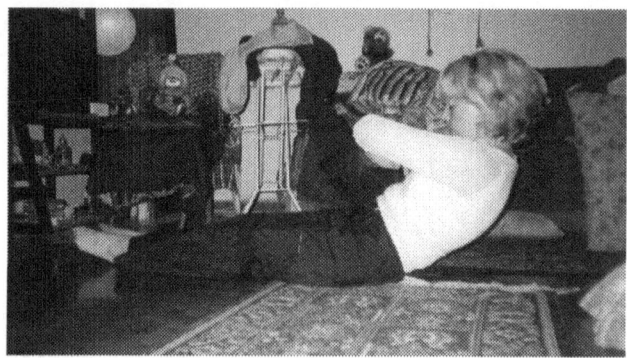

Fig. 1

4. Bring your arms out to your sides in a straight line with your shoulders so that your palms are looking at the back wall
5. Take the arms up to the ceiling keeping them next to the ears, then dive forward over your stretched legs
6. Bring the torso back to the original position and repeat the sequence 3 times

Benefits

Russian Curl initiates spinal alignment, works the shoulder in its socket and initiates the abdominal area.

The abdominals (abdomen) are four abdominal muscles in partitions:
1. The Transverse Abdominal muscles are the deepest of the four that force the air from the lungs, hence the exhale acquired whilst lifting is initiated in abdominal exercises
2. The Rectus Abdominal muscle functions to flex the trunk. We can see this movement done when the body is in the C-shape spine position on the mat
3. Internal and External Obliques work to rotate the trunk

Watchfulness

Do not hold your breath; a continuous inhale and exhale should be maintained throughout the exercise.

Try to keep your shoulders pressed away from your ears in order to eliminate the shrugging of shoulders.

You have just completed the Russian Curl exercise. Good work! Continue with The Spine Stretch Forward when you feel comfortable to continue.

**Important Note: All Stockpiles should begin with Stockpile Workout 1

<u>Stockpile Workout 9</u>

The Seal

Rowing

Spine Twists

The Saw

Russian Curl

Spine Stretch Forward

Spine Stretch Forward

<u>Technique</u>

1. Sit on the edge of your mat with your legs flexed out in front of you at shoulder width distance. Imagine your spine is supported by an imaginary wall

<u>Workout</u>

2. Bring your arms in front of you between your open legs and let the fingertips touch the floor. Begin walking those fingertips forward peeling the spine off an imaginary wall vertebrae by vertebrae

3. Walk the fingers back and re align your spine against the imaginary wall vertebrae by vertebrae

4. Repeat the sequence 3 more times

Benefits
The Spine Stretch Forward initiates spinal alignment and reduces Lordosis (inward curve of the lower back).

Watchfulness
Do not hold your breath; a continuous inhale and exhale should be maintained throughout the exercise.

Try to keep your shoulders pressed away from your ears in order to eliminate the shrugging of shoulders. Should you feel any tension in your lower back as you walk the fingers forward slightly bend the knees.

You have just completed the Spine Stretch Forward and Stockpile 9. Good work!

IMPROVEMENT RECORD STOCKPILE WORKOUT 9

The Seal

Rowing

Spine Twists

IMPROVEMENT RECORD STOCKPILE WORKOUT 9

The Saw

Russian Curl

Spine Stretch Forward

**Important Note: All Stockpiles should begin with Stockpile Workout 1
<u>Stockpile Workout 10</u>
The Arrow
The Diamond
Neck Roll
Planks
Leg Pull Back
The Swan Dive

The Arrow

<u>Technique & Workout—Level 1 (Fig. 1)</u>

1. Lie prone (on your stomach) with legs stretched out in a Pilates Stance. Bring the palms to rest on the side of your thighs
2. Squeeze the gluteus (buttocks), connect the shoulder blades and gently allow them to slide down your spine with chest resting on the mat and forehead looking down
3. Begin to walk those fingers towards your knees and feel the shoulders lower so that you obtain a long neck and the legs are stretching away from the torso
4. Rest then repeat 2 more times

<u>Technique—Level 2 (Fig. 1)</u>

5. Lie prone (on your stomach) with legs stretched out in a Pilates Stance. Bring the palms to rest on the side of your thighs
6. Squeeze the gluteus (buttocks), connect the shoulder blades and gently allow them to slide down your spine with chest resting on the mat and forehead looking down
7. Begin to walk those fingers towards your knees and feel the shoulders lower so that you obtain a long neck and the legs are stretching away from the torso

<u>Workout—Level 2</u>

8. Take the torso to twist gently to the right, bring it back to center then change the twist for the left side
9. Keep the technique in prime motion throughout the twist
10. Rest then repeat 2 more times

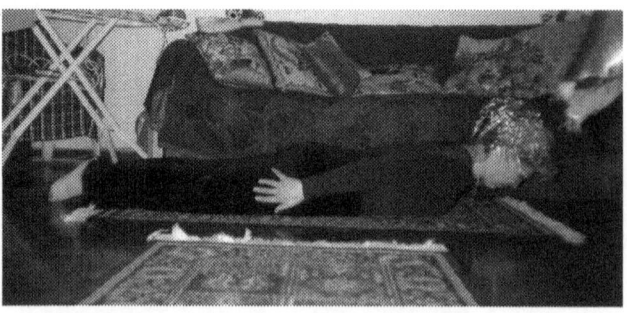

Fig. 1

Benefits

The Arrow initiates the elongation of the spinal cord separating the spinal disks from the vertebrae that are squeezed together due to gravity. It is entirely a technical exercise.

Watchfulness

Do not hold your breath; a continuous inhale and exhale should be maintained throughout the exercise.

Try to keep your shoulders pressed away from your ears in order to eliminate the shrugging of shoulders. Should you feel any tension in your lower back check to see if you are raising your chest off the mat; the chest should be in contact with the mat throughout the exercise.

You have just completed The Arrow. Good work! Continue with The Diamond when you feel comfortable to continue.

**Important Note: All Stockpiles should begin with Stockpile Workout 1

<u>Stockpile Workout 10</u>

The Arrow

The Diamond

Neck Roll

Planks

Leg Pull Back

The Swan Dive

The Diamond

<u>Technique</u>

1. Lie prone (on your stomach) with legs stretched out, shoulder width apart
2. Lift the upper body and bring the elbows under the shoulders to support the weight with palms in a prayer position

<u>Workout</u>

3. Squeeze the gluteus, connect the shoulder blades and gently allow them to slide down your spine. The forehead is looking diagonally forward
4. Feel the shoulders lower so that you obtain a long neck

<u>Important note:</u>

Two-fingers below the belly button is the center of your body. Imagine pressing this section towards your spine in order to eliminate the lower back from demolishing

5. Rest then repeat 2 more times

Benefits
The Diamond initiates the elongation of the spinal cord separating the spinal disks from the vertebrae that are squeezed together due to gravity. It also initiates the opening of the chest.

Watchfulness
Do not hold your breath; a continuous inhale and exhale should be maintained throughout the exercise.

Try to keep your shoulders pressed away from your ears in order to eliminate the shrugging of shoulders. Should you feel any tension in your lower back take those elbows forward into a diamond shape to alleviate any additional tension.

You have just completed The Diamond. Good work! Continue with the Neck Roll when you feel comfortable to continue.

**Important Note: All Stockpiles should begin with Stockpile Workout 1

Stockpile Workout 10

The Arrow

The Diamond

Neck Roll

Planks

Leg Pull Back

The Swan Dive

Neck Roll

Technique

1. Lie prone (on your stomach) with legs stretched out to shoulder width apart
2. Bring the palms to rest on the mat next to your chest and bend the elbows. Keep the elbows glued to your sides. This gives the arms a 90-degree angle (Fig. 1)

Workout

3. Squeeze the gluteus (buttocks), connect the shoulder blades and turn the head to look to the left shoulder. Try to gaze behind you
4. Take the head into a deep roll as the chin touches the surface of the chest until your head now looks to the other side of your shoulder. Try to gaze behind you

Important note:

Two-fingers below the belly button is the center of your body. Imagine pressing this section towards your spine in order to eliminate the lower back from demolishing

5. Repeat the roll 3 times to each side

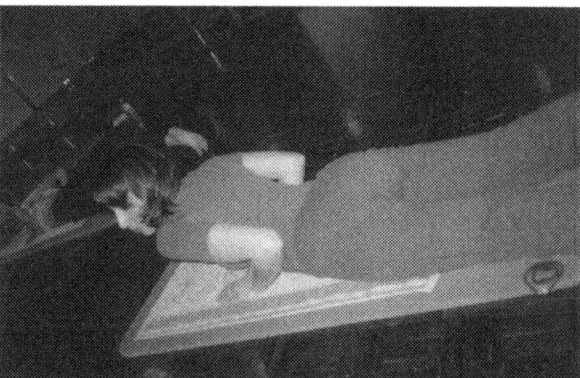

Fig. 1

Benefits

The Neck Roll initiates the elongation of the spinal cord separating the spinal disks from the vertebrae that are squeezed together due to gravity. It also initiates opening of the chest and helps release tension in the neck.

Watchfulness

Do not hold your breath; a continuous inhale and exhale should be maintained throughout the exercise.

Try to keep your shoulders pressed away from your ears in order to eliminate the shrugging of shoulders. Should you feel any tension in your lower back lower the torso to alleviate any additional tension.

You have just completed The Neck Roll. Good work! Continue with the Planks when you feel comfortable to continue.

**Important Note: All Stockpiles should begin with Stockpile Workout 1

<u>Stockpile Workout 10</u>

The Arrow

The Diamond

Neck Roll

Planks

Leg Pull Back

The Swan Dive

Planks

<u>Technique—Level 1</u>

1. Lie prone (on your stomach) with toes pressed into the mat
2. Raise the upper body bringing the elbows under the shoulders and palms in a prayer position
3. Squeeze the gluteus, connect the shoulder blades and gently allow them to slide down your spine. Keep the forehead looking to the floor

   <u>Important note:</u>

   Two-fingers below the belly button is the center of your body. Imagine pressing this section towards your spine in order to eliminate the lower back from demolishing

   <u>Workout—Level 1</u>
4. Begin to raise onto your knees (Fig. 1)

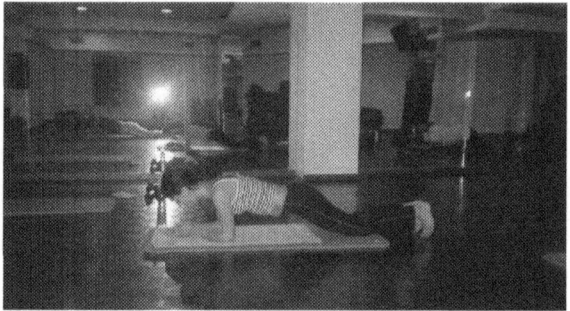

Fig. 1

5. Hold the position for 10 counts if possible. Keep the pelvis, back and head in one straight line with the floor

   <u>Technique—Level 2</u>
6. Lie prone (on your stomach) with legs stretched out shoulder width apart
7. Raise the upper body bringing the elbows under the shoulders and palms in a prayer position
8. Squeeze the gluteus, connect the shoulder blades and gently allow them to slide down your spine. Keep the forehead looking to the floor

   <u>Important note:</u>
9. Two-fingers below the belly button is the center of your body. Imagine pressing this section towards your spine in order to eliminate the lower back from demolishing

10. Try to straighten the legs for 10 counts (Fig. 2). Keep the pelvis, back and head in one straight line with the floor

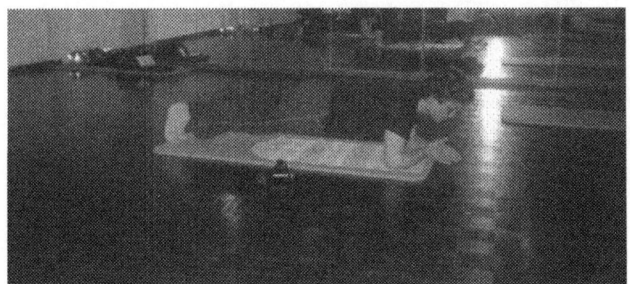

Fig. 2

Benefits
The Planks are complete body workouts.

Watchfulness
Do not hold your breath; a continuous inhale and exhale should be maintained throughout the exercise.

Try not to demolish the body weight onto the shoulders. Should you feel any tension in your lower back remain with level 1 of the exercise to alleviate any additional tension.

When in level 1 or 2, keep the pelvis, spine and head in one straight line with the floor.

You have just completed the Planks. Good work! Continue with the Leg Pull Back when you feel comfortable to continue.

**Important Note: All Stockpiles should begin with Stockpile Workout 1
<u>Stockpile Workout 10</u>
The Arrow
The Diamond
Neck Roll
Planks
Leg Pull Back
The Swan Dive

Leg Pull Back

<u>Technique</u>
1. Come onto your hands and knees with palms under the shoulders
2. Stretch the legs so that your pelvis, spine and head are in one straight line with the floor keeping the forehead facing the mat

<u>Workout</u>
3. Raise one leg flexed to bodyline (Fig. 1). Point the toe and lower the leg again.
4. Repeat 3 times alternating leg change

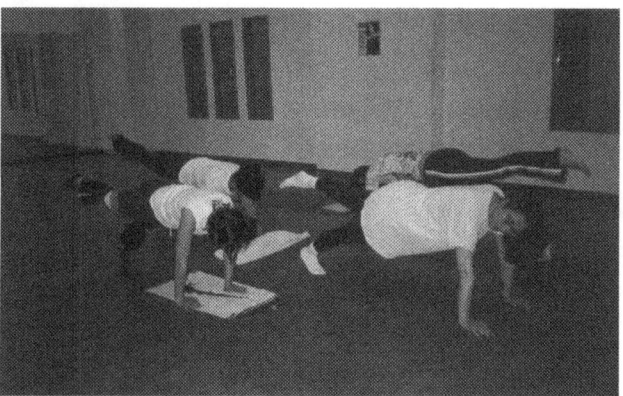

Fig. 1

Benefits
The Leg Pull Back is a complete body workout.

Watchfulness
Do not hold your breath; a continuous inhale and exhale should be maintained throughout the exercise.

Try not to demolish the body weight onto the shoulders. Should you feel any tension in your lower back do the exercise with knees on the mat to alleviate any additional tension.

Keep the pelvis, spine and head in one straight line.

You have just completed the Leg Pull Back. Good work! Continue with The Swan Dive when you feel comfortable to continue.

**Important Note: All Stockpiles should begin with Stockpile Workout 1
<u>Stockpile Workout 10</u>
The Arrow
The Diamond
Neck Roll
Planks
Leg Pull Back
The Swan Dive

The Swan Dive

<u>Technique</u>
1.   Lie on your stomach and stretch the legs behind you to shoulder width
2.   Bring the palms to rest on the mat beside your chest
<u>Workout</u>
3.   Begin to push up your upper body (Fig. 1a) and inhale. Roll onto your stomach and dive taking the arms forward and raising the legs behind you (Fig 1b). Exhale
4.   Roll back up to Fig. 1a position (inhale) and dive again (exhale)
5.   Repeat the dive 3-5 times

Fig. 1a

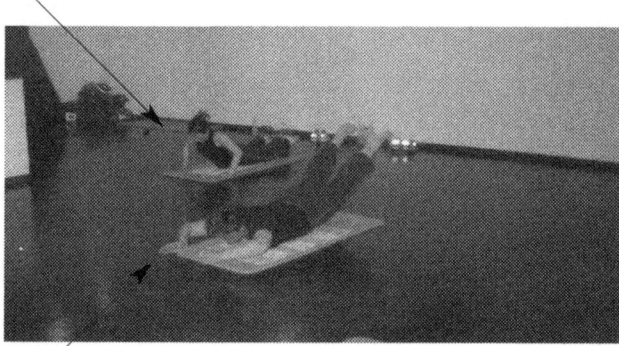

Fig. 1b

Benefits
The Swan Dive is a complete non-impact aerobic body workout.

Watchfulness
Do not hold your breath; a continuous inhale on the roll up and exhale on the dive should be maintained throughout the exercise.

Try to release the body when diving forward always rolling freely on the stomach for extra thrust. Should you feel any tension in your lower back do the exercise slowly for 3 repetitions only to alleviate any additional tension.

You have just completed the Swan Dive and Stockpile 10. Good work!

IMPROVEMENT RECORD STOCKPILE WORKOUT 10

The Arrow

The Diamond

Neck Roll

IMPROVEMENT RECORD STOCKPILE WORKOUT 10

Planks

Leg Pull Back

The Swan Dive

**Important Note: All Stockpiles should begin with Stockpile Workout 1
<u>Stockpile Workout 11</u>
Push-Up
Cat Legs
The Bear
Swimming
Breast Stroke

Push-Ups

<u>Technique</u>
1. Stand up and take those legs into a Pilates Stance. Zip up the inner thighs
2. Gently bend the knees and dive forward till your fingertips or palms touch the mat
3. Walk the hands four paces in front of you where your palms will now be under your shoulders, the pelvis and spine will be in one straight line (Fig. 1)

<u>Workout</u>
4. Bend the elbows for 3 small bends then straighten the arms
5. Repeat the arm sequence 2 more times
6. Walk the hands back towards your legs, and slowly rebuild the spine on the imaginary wall vertebrae by vertebrae until you are once again in standing position

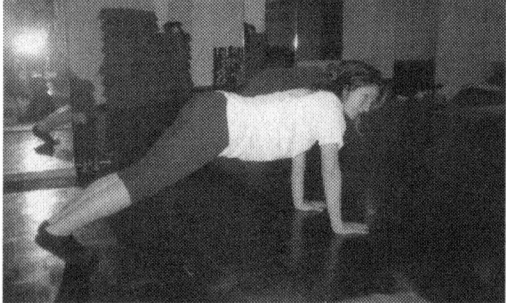

Fig. 1

Arabesque Push-Up

<u>Technique—Level 1</u>
1. Come onto your hands and knees in cat position with palms under the shoulders
2. Keep your elbows towards your sides

<u>Workout—Level 1</u>
3. Bend the elbows to lower the upper body horizontally towards the mat (Fig. 1). Do not allow the elbows to touch the mat. Straighten the arms to come back up

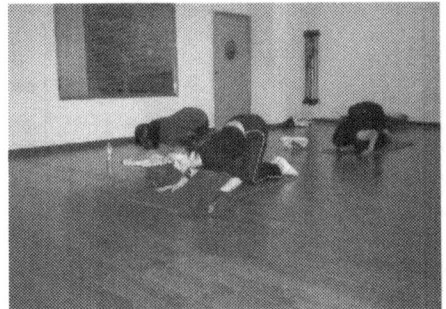

Fig. 1

Technique—Level 2

4.   Come onto your hands and knees in cat position with palms under the shoulders
5.   Keep your elbows towards your sides

Workout—Level 2

6.   Take the right leg up to an arabesque behind you (Fig. 2)

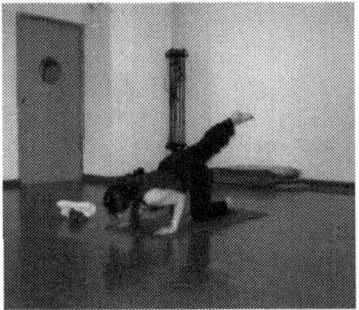

Fig. 2

7.   Bend the elbows to lower the upper body forward towards the mat. Straighten the arms to come back to the initial position

Benefits

The Push-Ups are complete body workouts and tones the triceps. When great force is initiated on the shoulder, it is vital that the scapula (shoulder blade) is fixed in place and kept against the ribcage.

Watchfulness

Do not hold your breath; a continuous inhale and exhale should be maintained throughout the exercise. Should you feel any tension in your lower back whilst doing this exercise, keep the knees on the mat to alleviate any additional tension and remain on Level 1 to give your body time to strengthen.

You have just completed the Push-Ups. Good work! Continue with Cat Legs when you feel comfortable to continue.

**Important Note: All Stockpiles should begin with Stockpile Workout 1
<u>Stockpile Workout 11</u>
Push-Up
Cat Legs
The Bear (Yoga Asana)
Swimming
Breast Stroke

Cat Legs
<u>Technique</u>
1.   Come onto your hands and knees in cat position with palms under the shoulders
2.   Take the right leg up to an arabesque behind you (Fig. 1)

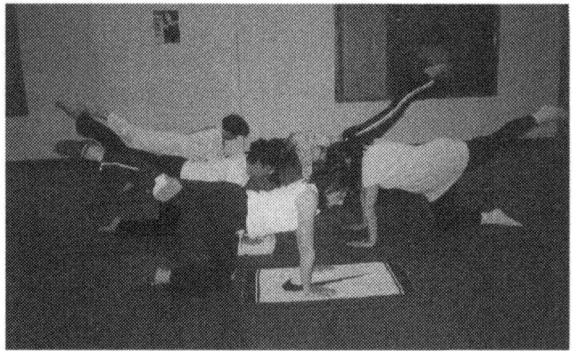

Fig. 1
<u>Workout</u>
3.   Bring that raised leg to your side to touch the floor (Fig. 2) take it behind you into the arabesque again.

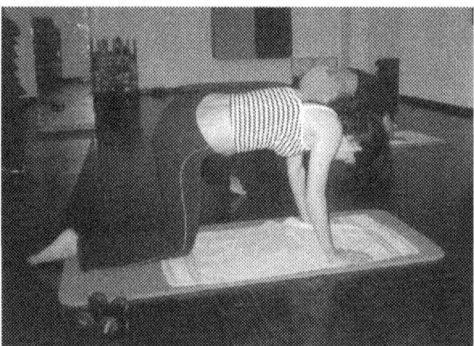

Fig. 2
4.   Repeat 10 times with each leg

Benefits
The Cat Legs initiates the buttocks, hips and strengthens the hip in its socket.

When great force is initiated on the shoulder, it is vital that the scapula (shoulder blade) is fixed in place and kept against the ribcage.

Watchfulness
Do not hold your breath; a continuous inhale and exhale should be maintained throughout the exercise.

Should you feel any tension in your lower back whilst doing the exercise, rest the elbows onto the mat to alleviate any additional tension.

You have just completed the Cat Legs. Good work! Continue with The Bear (Yoga Asana) when you feel comfortable to continue.

**Important Note: All Stockpiles should begin with Stockpile Workout 1

Stockpile Workout 11

Push-Up

Cat Legs

The Bear (Yoga Asana)

Swimming

Breast Stroke

The Bear

Technique

1. Come onto your hands and knees in cat position with palms under the shoulders
2. Raise the knees off the mat just enough to allow a sheet of paper to pass under

   Workout
3. Take the whole body back in a horizontal motion with a small range of motion, come back to the original position and repeat 2 more times before resting

Benefits
The Bear (Yoga Asana) initiates the quadriceps.

Watchfulness
Do not hold your breath; a continuous inhale and exhale should be maintained throughout the exercise.

You have just completed The Bear (Yoga Asana). Good work! Continue with the Swimming when you feel comfortable to continue.

**Important Note: All Stockpiles should begin with Stockpile Workout 1
<u>Stockpile Workout 11</u>
Push-Up
Cat Legs
The Bear (Yoga Asana)
Swimming
Breast Stroke

Swimming
<u>Technique</u>
1.   Lie in a prone position (on your stomach) with forehead facing the mat, legs stretched out behind you at shoulder width, and bring the arms to stretch out in front of you a little wider than shoulder width
<u>Workout</u>
2.   Raise the arms and legs without raising the chest off the mat and begin to alternate arms and legs as though swimming in the water
3.   Repeat for 10 counts each side before resting

Benefits
The Swimming initiates the Back muscles and spinal column.

Watchfulness
Do not hold your breath; a continuous inhale and exhale should be maintained throughout the exercise.

You have just completed the Swimming. Good work! Continue with the Breaststroke when you feel comfortable to continue.

**Important Note: All Stockpiles should begin with Stockpile Workout 1

<u>Stockpile Workout 11</u>

Push-Up

Cat Legs

The Bear (Yoga Asana)

Swimming

Breast Stroke

Breast Stroke

<u>Technique</u>

1. Lie in a prone position (on your stomach) with forehead facing the mat, legs stretched out behind you at shoulder width apart, and bring the palms to rest on the mat next to your chest

   <u>Workout</u>

2. Stretch the arms forward bringing them next to your ears. Inhale and take the arms back behind you. Exhale. Bring the arms back to their original position next to your chest—imagine your are swimming in a breaststroke motion in water

3. Do not allow the chest to raise off the mat to alleviate any tension in the lower back

4. Repeat the sequence for 10 counts before resting

Benefits

The Breast Stroke initiates the Back muscles and spinal column.

Watchfulness

Do not hold your breath; a continuous inhale on the stretch forward of the arms and exhale on bringing them next to your chest again should be maintained throughout the exercise.

You have just completed the Breast Stroke and Stockpile 11. Good work!

IMPROVEMENT RECORD STOCKPILE WORKOUT 11

Push-Up

Cat Legs

The Bear (Yoga Asana)

IMPROVEMENT RECORD STOCKPILE WORKOUT 11

Swimming

Breast Stroke

<u>Stockpile Workout 12</u>
Upside Down Table
Shoulder Lifts
Dead Zone

The cool-down allows you to take some time off for yourself. You are giving so many hours to other people that sometimes you usually forget to take some time for yourself, which you deserve. So let others wait, take these few moments for you to release and relax.

Upside Down Table
1. Lie relaxed in a supine position (on your back)
2. Raise your legs and arms towards the ceiling and feel the shoulders, spine and pelvis resting on the floor
3. Keep the legs and arms relaxed in the air and breath normally
4. When you feel you want to lower go ahead and do so

Shoulder Lifts
1. Lie relaxed in a supine position (on your back)
2. Bring the knees to bend in a 90-degree angle with soles on the floor
3. Raise the arms towards the ceiling and feel the shoulders, spine and pelvis resting on the floor
4. Take the right arm and imagine you want to touch the ceiling with the fingertips
5. Notice the right shoulder blade raise from the mat
6. Gently bring the shoulder blade back to the mat and change arms
7. Complete 3 sequences to each arm before relaxing

Dead Zone
1. Lie relaxed in a supine position completely flat on the mat (you can bend the legs if this position feels uncomfortable in your lower back to reduce tension)
2. Connect the heels and then allow the feet to drop out in a natural position
3. Bring the arms next to you slightly away from the body with palms facing up. Relax the arms, shoulders, hips, and legs
4. You may close your eyes for extra relaxation
5. Think of your entire body weight relaxing to the floor
6. Mentally soften each part of the body beginning from the toes, moving up to the ankles, calves, knees, thighs, and relaxing the pelvis
7. Mentally soften the spine to release vertebrae by vertebrae
8. Soften the shoulders, the arms, the elbows, the wrists, and even the center of the palms soften and release
9. Inhale softly and exhale softly feeling the chest and ribcage release
10. Soften the muscles on the face allowing the lips to part and forehead to relax
11. Gently allow the head to roll on its axel to the right with its own weight and always in contact with the floor. Let it roll back to center and slowly to the other side

12. Feel the neck release as the head rolls on its axel to center again
13. Remain here for as long as you feel comfortable

You deserved that. Well done!

NOTES

PILATES BABY STOCKPILES

*Important Note: All Pilates Baby Stockpiles should begin with Stockpile Workout 1

<u>Pilates Baby Stockpile 1</u>

Neck Roll

Swan Dive

Neck Roll—Swan Dive (For full technique and what to be aware of, look at these exercises in their Stockpile Workouts)

<u>Technique</u>

1. Lie prone (on your stomach) with legs stretched out to shoulder width
2. Bring the palms next to your chest and bend the elbows. Keep the elbows glued to your sides. This gives the arms a 90-degree angle

<u>Workout</u>

3. Squeeze the gluteus (buttocks), connect the shoulder blades and turn the head to look to the left shoulder. Try to gaze behind you
4. Roll the head allowing the chin to brush the surface of your chest until your head now looks to the other side. Try to gaze behind you
5. Roll the head allowing the chin to brush the surface of your chest until your head now looks to the other side. Try to gaze behind you
6. Look straight ahead for the Swan Dive
7. Roll onto your stomach as though you are diving into water taking the arms forward and raising the legs behind you. Exhale
8. Roll back up, catch your self with your arms then dive again stretching the arms forward bringing them next to your ears
9. Repeat the sequence 3 times

NOTES

*Important Note: All Pilates Baby Stockpiles should begin with Stockpile Workout 1

Pilates Baby Stockpile 2

Hip Circles

Can-Can

Hip Circles—Can-Can (For full technique and what to be aware of, look at these exercises in their Stockpile Workouts)

<u>Technique</u>

1.   Sit up on your mat and take those arms behind you for support. If you have a delicate lower back, rest on the elbows
2.   Turn the hip to the right then stretch the legs diagonally in a Pilates Stance. This will bring the legs to a diagonal 45-degree angle

<u>Workout</u>

3.   Draw a big circle with those legs to the right and circle around to the left side. Try not to bend the legs as you lower; keep control
4.   Draw a big circle with those legs to the left and circle around to the right side. Try not to bend the legs as you lower; keep control
5.   Staying on the right side, draw 6 small circles with the toes
6.   Draw again a big circle with those legs to the right and circle around to the left side, then staying on the left side, draw 6 small circles with the toes
7.   Draw a big circle with those legs to the left and circle around to the right side. Try not to bend the legs as you lower; keep control
8.   Repeat 3 times each side

NOTES

*Important Note: All Pilates Baby Stockpiles should begin with Stockpile Workout 1

Pilates Baby Stockpile 3

Side Isometric Level 1

Chest Expansion

Side Isometric Level 1—Chest Expansion (For full technique and what to be aware of, look at these exercises in their Stockpile Workouts)

Technique

1. Sit onto your right hip and bring your right palm to the floor. Have the palm placed under the shoulder line
2. Come on up on your right knee and have it placed in line with the hip joint

Workout

3. Bring your left arm to stretch to the ceiling with palm facing forward. Try to get both arms to form one straight line
4. Hold position for 5 counts then come to a kneeling position with both knees on the floor, thighs looking forward
5. Bring those arms by your side, palms facing back
6. Stretch the arms towards the back wall and feel how your chest expands
7. Turn the head to look to your right then turn your head to your left then bring it back to center again bringing your arms by your sides to rest
8. Change sides for the Side Isometric then continue with the Chest Expansion again
9. Repeat once to each side

NOTES

*Important Note: All Pilates Baby Stockpiles should begin with Stockpile Workout 1

Pilates Baby Stockpile 4

Chest Expansion

The Mermaid

Chest Expansion—The Mermaid (For full technique and what to be aware of, look at these exercises in their Stockpile Workouts)

<u>Technique</u>

1. Come to a kneeling position with both knees on the floor, thighs looking forward
2. Bring those arms by your side, palms facing back

<u>Workout</u>

3. Stretch the arms towards the back wall and feel how your chest expands
4. Turn your head to look to your right then turn your head to your left then center again and bring your arms by your sides to go to The Mermaid Level 1
5. Sit on your right hip side. Bend those legs and take them to the left side of your body. This will bring the legs to a 90-degree angle
6. Grasp your left ankle with your left hand for support and take your right hand to stretch towards the ceiling next to your ear. Try to lower the shoulder from the ear to avoid the shrugging motion
7. Straighten the spine by connecting the shoulder blades together and sliding them down your spine (depress). Imagine you are sitting against an imaginary wall
8. Bend your torso to the left side towards the ankles and feel the stretch on your right side. You are now in the Mermaid position
9. Hold this position for 5 inhales and 5 exhales
10. Come back to neutral position
11. Come onto your knees for the Chest Expansion again and then go into The Mermaid exercise on the other side
12. Repeat once to each side

NOTES

*Important Note: All Pilates Baby Stockpiles should begin with Stockpile Workout 1
Pilates Baby Stockpile 5
Pilates Lunges
Back Curtsey Lunges

Pilates Lunges—Back Curtsey Lunges

<u>Technique</u>

1. Come to a third dance position (the right heel touches the inside of the left foot; Your right knee should be looking to the right)

    <u>Workout</u>

2. Take the right leg out diagonally in a wide stance and lower the hips to come into a lunge position. This will bring the bent leg in a 90-degree angle

    <u>Important Note:</u>

    Do not allow the knee to go beyond the toes; keep the knee in line with the ankle

3. Allow the back leg to stretch out with your foot and heel on the floor

4. Bring both arms to stretch in front of you next to your ears. The body now is in one straight diagonal line from the fingers down to the heel of the back leg

5. Hold position for 5 counts then push up from your right bent leg and take the leg diagonally behind you, do a curtsey taking the body down

6. Push up and come to standing third dance position

7. Repeat 3 times with each leg

NOTES

*Important Note: All Pilates Baby Stockpiles should begin with Stockpile Workout 1 (For full technique and what to be aware of, look at these exercises in their Stockpile Workouts)
Pilates Baby Stockpile 6
Scissors I, II

Scissors I, II

Technique I

1. Lie in a supine position (on your back) and stretch your legs towards the ceiling in a Pilates Stance. This will have the legs in a 90-degree angle
2. Begin by raising the head off the mat and imagine you are holding a small tennis ball between your chin and sternum (chest). This will allow for a long neck. The shoulders are now in a 35-degree angle off the mat

Workout I

3. Take one leg towards your face and the other leg stretch towards the floor without letting it touch the mat. Hold the ankles
4. Pulse the leg towards your face for 2 counts and simultaneously pulse the leg towards the floor for 2 counts
5. Switch legs. Inhale on one switch and exhale on the other switch
6. Repeat the sequence and alternate for 10 switches with each leg

Workout II

7. Do the Scissors without holding the legs. Keep the arms by your side just above the mat with elbows slightly bent and begin to scissor those legs through the air

Important Note:

Should you feel that your lower back is lifting from the mat, bend the legs slightly and do a smaller movement with the scissors or you can always grasp the legs again as in Workout I. Do whatever makes you feel comfortable

NOTES

*Important Note: All Pilates Baby Stockpiles should begin with Stockpile Workout 1 (For full technique and what to be aware of, look at these exercises in their Stockpile Workouts)

Pilates Baby Stockpile 7

Ballerina One

The Ball

Ballerina One—The Ball

Technique—Ballerina One

1.   Sit cross-legged. Imagine your spine is supported against a wall. Bend those arms so that the elbows are looking out to the sides and palms facing your chest. This will bring the elbow to a 45-degree angle

Workout—Ballerina One

2.   Take the arms back to connect the shoulder blades (adduction) and your elbows are looking at the back wall

3.   Slide those arms down your side and feel the shoulder blades slide down (depress). The elbows are now looking to the mat

4.   Raise the bent arms over your head with palms looking down at the top of your head

5.   To end the Ballerina bring the arms back to their original position and repeat 2 more times

6.   Go straight to The Ball exercise

Technique—The Ball

7.   Sit on the edge of your mat with your legs bent to the chest and gently grasp your ankles. The right hand on the left ankle and the left hand on the right ankle

8.   Open the legs slightly to allow your head to pass through. Stay curled up like a ball

9.   Tilt back slightly to balance on your sit bones with tiptoes touching the mat

Workout—The Ball

10.   Keep your head in whilst you begin to roll onto the spine vertebrae by vertebrae then roll back up like a ball

11.   Repeat the ball exercise for 5 rolls

Important note:

Stop the roll of the spine at the shoulder blades and never onto the neck area

NOTES

STANDING SERIES

*Important Note: Standing Series exercises should begin with Stockpile Workout 1

<u>Standing Series</u>

1. Biceps I, II
2. Triceps
3. The Bug
4. Chest Expansion
5. The Boxer
6. The Zipper
7. Shaving the Head
8. Arm Circles
9. Standing Wall Peeling the Spine
10. Standing Chair
11. Standing Cool Down

Biceps I, II

<u>Technique—I</u>

1. Stand in a Pilates Stance holding 2.2 lb (1kg) weights
2. Raise the arms to shoulder height straight out in front of you and turn the arms outwards so the weights face the ceiling
   <u>Workout—I</u>
3. Begin to bend the arms at the elbows bringing the weights towards you then stretch the arms out again keeping the elbows steady at shoulder height
4. Repeat for 10
   <u>Technique II</u>
5. After your repetitions take the arms out to the side at shoulder height where the weights are still facing the ceiling
   <u>Workout II</u>
6. Begin to bend the arms at the elbows bringing the weights towards your shoulders then stretch the arms out again keeping the elbows steady at shoulder height
7. Repeat for 10

NOTES

*Important Note: Standing Series exercises should begin with Stockpile Workout 1

<u>Standing Series</u>

1. Biceps I, II
2. Triceps
3. The Bug
4. Chest Expansion
5. The Boxer
6. The Zipper
7. Shaving the Head
8. Arm Circles
9. Standing Wall Peeling the Spine
10. Standing Chair
11. Standing Cool Down

Triceps

<u>Technique</u>

1. Stand with legs at shoulder width holding 2.2 lb (1kg) weights
2. Bend forward so the upper body is now in one straight line with the floor

   <u>Important Note:</u>

   Should your lower back feel uncomfortable, gently bend the knees
3. Bring your arms to your sides and bend the elbows gluing them to your ribs. The weights are looking in towards you

   <u>Workout</u>
4. Straighten the arms back to the height of your upper body and bend again to original position. Try not to move the elbows or upper body whilst doing this movement; control. Repeat 10 times

NOTES

*Important Note: Standing Series exercises should begin with Stockpile Workout 1

<u>Standing Series</u>

1. Biceps I, II
2. Triceps
3. The Bug
4. Chest Expansion
5. The Boxer
6. The Zipper
7. Shaving the Head
8. Arm Circles
9. Standing Wall Peeling the Spine
10. Standing Chair
11. Standing Cool Down

The Bug

<u>Technique</u>

1. Stand with legs at shoulder width holding 2.2 lb (1kg) weights
2. Bend forward so the upper body is now in one straight line with the floor
   <u>Important Note:</u>
   Should your lower back feel uncomfortable, gently bend the knees
3. Bring the weights in front of the chest so your elbows are looking to the sides and your arms are shaped in a circle
   <u>Workout</u>
4. Take the arms out and back so the elbows are now looking to the ceiling. Try not to let the upper body move whilst doing this and feel the shoulder blades connect
5. Bring the arms again to original position with weights in front of the chest
6. Repeat 10 times

NOTES

*Important Note: Standing Series exercises should begin with Stockpile Workout 1

Standing Series

1. Biceps I, II
2. Triceps
3. The Bug
4. Chest Expansion
5. The Boxer
6. The Zipper
7. Shaving the Head
8. Arm Circles
9. Standing Wall Peeling the Spine
10. Standing Chair
11. Standing Cool Down

Chest Expansion

Technique

1. Stand in a Pilates Stance holding 2.2 lb (1kg) weights
2. Bring those arms by your side, palms facing back

Workout

3. Stretch the arms backwards towards the back wall and feel how your chest expands
4. Turn your head to look to your right then turn the head to look to your left then bring the head centre again and bring your arms by your sides
5. Repeat 5 times

NOTES

*Important Note: Standing Series exercises should begin with Stockpile Workout 1

Standing Series

1. Biceps I, II
2. Triceps
3. The Bug
4. Chest Expansion
5. The Boxer
6. The Zipper
7. Shaving the Head
8. Arm Circles
9. Standing Wall Peeling the Spine
10. Standing Chair
11. Standing Cool Down

The Boxer

Technique

1. Stand with legs at shoulder width holding 2.2 lb (1kg) weights
2. Bend forward so the upper body is now in one straight line with the floor

   Important Note:

   Should your lower back feel uncomfortable, gently bend the knees

   Workout
3. Stretch your right arm forward next to your ear with weight facing the floor and stretch your left arm backwards bringing it next to your hip with weight facing the ceiling
4. Now bend both arms at the elbows bringing them next to your ribs with elbows facing the ceiling
5. Switch to bring your left arm stretched forward next to your ear with weight facing the floor and stretch your right arm backwards next to your hip with weight facing the ceiling
6. Continue doing this switch for another 5 repetitions

NOTES

*Important Note: Standing Series exercises should begin with Stockpile Workout 1

Standing Series

1. Biceps I, II
2. Triceps
3. The Bug
4. Chest Expansion
5. The Boxer
6. The Zipper
7. Shaving the Head
8. Arm Circles
9. Standing Wall Peeling the Spine
10. Standing Chair
11. Standing Cool Down

The Zipper

Technique

1. Stand in a Pilates Stance holding 2.2 lb (1kg) weights

   Workout

2. Your arms are in front of you with palms looking in. Bend the elbows so the arms raise bringing the weights to chest level

3. Take the arms back down again. Imagine you are zipping up the front of your coat and zipping it back down again

4. Do a repetition of 10

NOTES

*Important Note: Standing Series exercises should begin with Stockpile Workout 1

<u>Standing Series</u>

1. Biceps I, II
2. Triceps
3. The Bug
4. Chest Expansion
5. The Boxer
6. The Zipper
7. Shaving the Head
8. Arm Circles
9. Standing Wall Peeling the Spine
10. Standing Chair
11. Standing Cool Down

Shaving the Head

<u>Technique</u>

1. Stand in a Pilates Stance holding 2.2 lb (1kg) weights
2. Stretch the arms up to the ceiling with weights facing forward

<u>Workout</u>

3. Bend at the elbows bringing the arms into a diamond shape and let the weights pass behind the head as though you are shaving the back of your head. Slightly tilt the torso forward to allow comfort of motion
4. Stretch arms up to the ceiling again
5. Repeat 10 times

NOTES

*Important Note: Standing Series exercises should begin with Stockpile Workout 1

<u>Standing Series</u>

1. Biceps I, II
2. Triceps
3. The Bug
4. Chest Expansion
5. The Boxer
6. The Zipper
7. Shaving the Head
8. Arm Circles
9. Standing Wall Peeling the Spine
10. Standing Chair
11. Standing Cool Down

Arm Circles

<u>Technique</u>

1. Stand in a Pilates Stance holding 2.2 lb (1kg) weights
2. Your arms in front of you slightly bent at the elbows to protect the shoulder in its socket

<u>Workout</u>

3. Begin to draw 4 upward small circles in the air in front of you with the right arm then draw 4 downward small circles in the air in front of you
4. Change arm so you now draw 4 upward small circles in the air in front of you with the left arm then draw 4 downward small circles in the air in front of you
5. Repeat 3 times with each arm
6. Now for both arms; draw 4 small circles outwards and upwards in the air in front of you then draw 4 inward and downward circles in the air in front of you
7. Repeat 3 times

NOTES

*Important Note: Standing Series exercises should begin with Stockpile Workout 1

<u>Standing Series</u>

1. Biceps I, II
2. Triceps
3. The Bug
4. Chest Expansion
5. The Boxer
6. The Zipper
7. Shaving the Head
8. Arm Circles
9. Standing Wall Peeling the Spine
10. Standing Chair
11. Standing Cool Down

Standing Wall Peeling the Spine

<u>Technique</u>

1. Stand against a wall. Heels together touching the wall, hips, spine and head against the wall

2. You will notice a small gap in your lower back. To eliminate this, take a small step forward and you will notice that the gap has diminished. Relax the shoulders and place the palms against the wall

   <u>Workout</u>

3. Begin to peel the spine vertebrae by vertebrae from the wall. Begin with the head, shoulders, back, lower back and let your head droop forward in this forward bend with arms dangling down to the floor

   <u>Important Note:</u>

   Should you feel any tension in your lower back slightly bend your knees to eliminate this tension

4. Now roll the spine back up to the wall vertebrae by vertebrae till you are standing once again against the wall with your whole body touching

NOTES

*Important Note: Standing Series exercises should begin with Stockpile Workout 1

<u>Standing Series</u>

1. Biceps I, II
2. Triceps
3. The Bug
4. Chest Expansion
5. The Boxer
6. The Zipper
7. Shaving the Head
8. Arm Circles
9. Standing Wall Peeling the Spine
10. Standing Chair
11. Standing Cool Down

Standing Chair

<u>Technique</u>

1. Stand against a wall and bring your legs to shoulder width. You will need to take the legs forward in front of you away from the wall

<u>Workout</u>

2. Slowly slide your back down the wall and come into a chair position. This will bring your legs to bend at the knees into a 90-degree angle

<u>Important Note:</u>

Do not allow the knees to fall forward keep them over your ankles and never allow the pelvis to drop lower than the knees

3. Raise your arms in front of you, chest height, then stretch them over your head so the back of the palms are against the wall

4. Slide back up to standing position. Repeat the Standing Chair 3 times

NOTES

*Important Note: Standing Series exercises should begin with Stockpile Workout 1

<u>Standing Series</u>

1. Biceps I, II
2. Triceps
3. The Bug
4. Chest Expansion
5. The Boxer
6. The Zipper
7. Shaving the Head
8. Arm Circles
9. Standing Wall Peeling the Spine
10. Standing Chair
11. Standing Cool Down

Standing Cool Down

1. Stand up with legs in second position ballet. This would be legs at shoulder width with knees and toes turned out

2. Keep the knees soft then gently roll forward to scoop the body down and arms to pass through those legs

    <u>Important Note:</u>

    Should you feel any tension in your lower back whilst rolling forward, gently bend those knees to alleviate any additional tension

3. Roll back up to standing position and do the forward scoop to the right side. Roll back up to standing position and do the forward scoop to the left side

4. Roll back up then keeping the legs firmly glued in that third position ballet turn your whole body so it twists towards the right.

5. Your torso is now facing the back leg; allow the twist to initiate on the ball of your foot. Keep your right leg facing right and your left leg stretched out behind you

6. Scoop forward towards your back leg as far as you can and hold with control

7. Come out of the twist to initial forward position and change side

NOTES

ATHLETIC TAI-CHI STOCKPILES

*Important Note: Athletic Tai-Chi Exercises should begin with Stockpile Workout 1

<u>Athletic Tai-Chi Stockpile 1</u>
Abduction
Parting Horse's Rein

Abduction

<u>Technique</u>
1.   Stand next to a wall for support with the right side facing it and put your right hand against the wall with a slightly bent elbow
2.   Stand with feet shoulder width then turn the right leg to face the wall. In other words your knee faces the wall. This allows for the pelvis to remain open whilst doing the exercise
3.   Flex the left leg and slightly turn the toes to look inwards
      <u>Workout</u>
4.   Raise the left flexed leg to hip level and return it back down again. If hip level feels too uncomfortable, you can always raise it to the height you feel comfortable
5.   Try to do 16 repetitions before taking a hip stretch
      <u>Hip Stretch</u>
6.   Come away from the wall and cross one leg over the other, bend forwards a little to allow for the stretch with hands on the thighs for support and then shift the hip towards the back leg. Change leg crossing and do the same stretch on the other side
7.   Go ahead and do the abduction exercise on the left side

NOTES

*Important Note: Athletic Tai-Chi Exercises should begin with Stockpile Workout 1

Athletic Tai-Chi Stockpile 1

Abduction

Parting Horse's Rein

Parting Horse's Rein

Technique

1. Shift into your right leg and feel the buoyancy of the right leg
2. Bring your hands in front of you close to your chest and imagine you are holding a small sphere. Your right palm is on top of the sphere

    Workout
3. Shift the left leg diagonally forward and simultaneously part the arms where your left arm extends towards the diagonal and your right arm goes towards your hip
4. Come back to the buoyancy position
5. Do 3 slow repetitions then go for 8 quicker movements
6. Switch sides.
7. As you progress, do 4 quicker movements to each side, then 2 quicker movements to each side and finally 8 single movements to each side

NOTES

*Important Note: Athletic Tai-Chi Exercises should begin with Stockpile Workout 1

Athletic Tai-Chi Stockpile 2

Repulse the Monkey

Horse Stance

Repulse the Monkey

<u>Technique</u>

1. Stand on your right leg and feel the buoyancy of the right leg. Take the left leg on tiptoe in front of you
2. Left arm stretched out in front of you with palm facing up and right arm bend behind you with palm facing forward

<u>Workout</u>

3. Take front leg behind you diagonally and turn the body in to press the back hand forward and the front hand back
4. Back to original position. Don't forget it's a diagonal movement and the twists should always be made on the balls of the feet
5. Do this in 3 slow repetitions
6. Keep the front leg behind you diagonally, turn the body in to press the back hand forward and the front hand back
7. Now just do the hand movements as you remain in leg position for as long as you are comfortable then change sides

NOTES

*Important Note: Athletic Tai-Chi Exercises should begin with Stockpile Workout 1

Athletic Tai-Chi Stockpile 2

Repulse the Monkey

Horse Stance

Horse Stance

Technique

1. Stand with legs in a wider stance than shoulder width
2. Bring your feet to look forward with knees slightly turned out. Try to keep the spine against an imaginary wall throughout this exercise

Workout

3. Begin to squat as though you are sitting in a chair and coming back up again. Take the squat as low as you feel comfortable but never below knee height. If you feel that you are leaning forward, reposition that spine against the wall again and continue
4. Try to do 8 single counts, then keep the squat low and pulse it out for 4 counts then return to your 8 single counts

Hip Stretch

Cross one leg over the other, bend forwards a little to allow for the stretch with hands on the thighs for support then shift the hip towards the back leg. Change leg crossing and do the same stretch on the other side

NOTES

0-595-31925-4